Praise for *You're N*

Zach does a great job of normalizing what mental health struggles. He humanizes an [illegible] college students experience but may be too shy to publicly express. A recommended read for those experiencing some kind of struggle or curious to learn more about brain and mental health.

—Nicholas T. Frias, director of fraternity and sorority life, Sacred Heart University

You're Not Alone points a bright light at topics too many are in the dark about: depression and anxiety. Westerbeck's writing style makes these incredibly hard and often shameful mental health issues feel less isolating and more approachable. I highly recommend this book if you or someone you know needs to feel a little less alone right now. It's an important read!

—James Robilotta, author of *Leading Imperfectly* and host of *Diner Talks with James*

Zach Westerbeck has produced an outstanding resource for the college student dealing with depression and anxiety. It is a must-read for both the struggling and the healthy mind. It offers hope and a path of light for those caught in a vortex of darkness.

—Louis M. Profeta, MD, LinkedIn Top Voice in Health Care and author of *The Patient in Room Nine Says He's God*

Prepare for your emotions to be validated, experiences normalized, and mind empowered. *You're Not Alone* is a compact guide to stepping into a healthier version of yourself.

—Christian N. Beck, LMHC, mental health counselor, Counseling and Psychological Services, Colgate University

This book is exactly what the world needs right now: a playbook for how to manage brain health and overcome anxiety and depression. Zach shares his powerful mental health story and the steps we can take to reach our full potential.

—Joseph Moheban, CEO and cofounder of 220 Leadership Academy

You're Not Alone is set up to provide personal experience, significant research on brain health, and great strategies and resources to help readers.

—Paul Ferrante, MA, assistant director of student engagement, NYIT

Zach Westerbeck has created an essential student resource for brain health that perfectly outlines every step of recovery. Zach's personal journey combined with his breadth of knowledge about brain health works directly to "smash the stigma." This book will serve as a lifeline for any student.

—Victorina Jeffers, Fraternity & Sorority Life Professional

Zach Westerbeck's book portrays the raw truth of what many men go through but never speak about. This book has opened up my eyes to urge other men to speak up about their issues and make men's mental health a topic of conversation. Thank you, Zach, for this realization, and thank you for being your authentic self with every word written in this book!

—Shiv Rad, author of *The Regular Effect*

Zach's book reminds young people that when the dark clouds of adversity gather, they are not alone and there is hope for the future. The messaging and thoughtfulness of each technique Zach presents will undoubtedly help college students who deal with anxiety and depression get the help they need. In the end, this book will help lead each reader to a happier and healthier tomorrow.

—Marcos Guzman, assistant dean of students, University of Arizona

Zach Westerbeck has curated a much-needed, approachable, and timely must-read for those looking to better understand, face, and conquer the struggles of mental wellness, substance reliance, and an ever-changing social landscape. While most specifically geared toward college-going young adults, any reader will find true value and points of connection with Zach's undeniably heartfelt, direct, and impactful words. As a professional who had worked in the mental health, substance and education space for nearly 20 years, I unequivocally endorse *You're Not Alone*!

—Daniel Patterson, founder and CEO of Patterson Perspective Inc.

Zach's words are powerful and relatable for any college student experiencing difficulties. He breaks down complex concepts in a way that is easily understandable. Zach equips the reader with a roadmap that includes a variety of practical options for recovery, and he emphasizes that everyone deserves to receive help. Every college student should be handed a copy of this book!

—Julia Broglie, founder of BroglieBox

Zach Westerbeck has created a resource that every college student should read. This book will help students who are struggling with anxiety and depression find the strength to get help and will also help students identify the early signs in their peers. He lays out a compelling framework for destigmatizing mental health challenges and having difficult mental health conversations. His personal story is powerful. Hopefully, many young people connect with it to find their own personal strength to get help and persevere.

—Robert Wilson, founding partner, Culture Shift Team

Zach has produced a book that can resonate with anyone who is struggling or has struggled with anxiety and depression and is looking for a way to create a healthy mind. His book provides relatable personal experiences as well as a thoughtful plan to assist his readers in breaking the stigma associated with mental health and seeing that there is light at the end of what seems like darkness. His book is a must-read!

—Brianna J. Davis, MSW, CEO and founder of Esperanza de Tejas, Inc.

YOU'RE NOT ALONE

IF YOU OR A LOVED ONE IS EXPERIENCING THOUGHTS OF SUICIDE OR IS IN NEED OF HELP, PLEASE CALL THE NATIONAL SUICIDE PREVENTION LIFELINE AT 1-800-273-TALK.

Zachary David Westerbeck

YOU'RE NOT ALONE

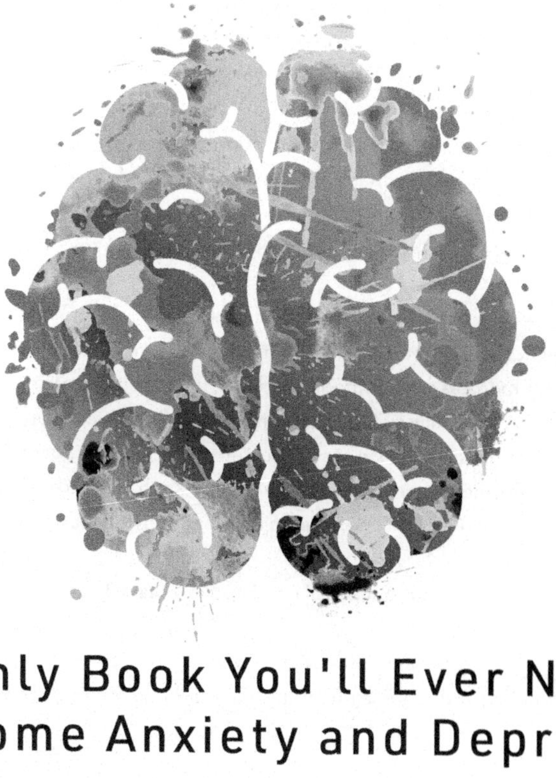

The Only Book You'll Ever Need to Overcome Anxiety and Depression

You're Not Alone: The Only Book You'll Ever Need to Overcome Anxiety and Depression

Zach Westerbeck is not a licensed medical professional. Zach Westerbeck is not trained in diagnosing psychological or medical conditions. Zach Westerbeck is not a substitute for medical care or medical advice. If you require assistance with any mental health or medical issue, please contact your health care provider for any medical care or medical advice. Zach Westerbeck makes no guarantees of any kind that the information or services provided by Zach Westerbeck will improve the client's situation and/or ensure admission into any educational institution.

Paperback ISBN: 978-0-578-75420-8

Cover and interior design by Liz Schrieter
Editing and book production by Reading List Editorial: readinglisteditorial.com

TO YOU. MAY YOU HEAL YOUR BRAIN SO YOU REALIZE YOUR FULLEST POTENTIAL.

CONTENTS

INTRODUCTION

Chances are, you're reading this book because you know what it feels like to be depressed or anxious—or both. So you probably know already how isolating, debilitating, frustrating, and exhausting anxiety and depression can feel. And if so, you're probably sick of feeling this way, and who wouldn't be? Anxiety and depression can be hugely disruptive, especially for someone who's got a lot on their plate, like you do. Between juggling a heavy course load, finding time to hang out with friends, and being involved in clubs, you are trying your very best. On top of all that, dealing with a pounding heart, racing thoughts, and feelings of deep sadness can make a lot feel like too much. Worst of all, you might feel like you can't share what you're going through with anyone, so besides a close friend or two, nobody seems to get you.

If you're feeling alone, scared, abnormal, or like a failure right now, I want you to know that I get you. I've felt that way, too. The truth is that you're not alone, and you're not a failure. No matter how much you're struggling in your classes. No matter how few friends you've made while on campus. No matter the traumas you've experienced with family. What you're dealing with is totally normal. In fact, it's so normal that thousands of college students across the country are having the same thoughts and feeling the exact same way as you do *right now.* Think about that.

So you know that voice inside your head that's always saying things like, "Why can't I get myself together!? Why am I so lazy? Why can't I be stronger and just push through? Why can't I stick to a routine? I'll probably always feel this way. I'm never going to have a normal life again"?

That voice is lying to you. You're having these thoughts because you're still trying to get a grasp on your anxiety and depression. Once those feelings become more manageable, everything else in your life will start to improve. I promise.

It's time to reclaim your life from anxiety and depression, and through the course of this book, you and I are going to work together to do just that. What you're going through is extremely normal, treatable, and things can get better. You just need the right tools and the right team.

About that team: I'm willing to bet that you've never seen a mental health professional before. If you have, my guess is that it was a one-time experience or only lasted a few appointments. You wouldn't be alone there, either. When they're going through a tough time, a lot of people try to handle it on their own. After all, seeking help for psychiatric challenges can be perceived as awkward or embarrassing, and in a lot of families and friend groups, discussing emotions can be taboo. So if you'd rather wait until things are as bad as they can possibly be before opening up to someone, I get it. I get it because I once waited until I didn't want to live anymore to seek help. I'll explain.

My Rock-Bottom Moment

One evening, back in the spring of 2016, I was standing on the balcony of my fourth-floor apartment, taking in the cotton-candy color of the North Carolina sky. As I leaned against the railing, looking out at the horizon and admiring how beautiful everything was, I happened to glance down at the parking lot, some forty feet below.

"You should just jump," I heard a voice in my mind say. My heart began to race. The voice continued, "If you jump from this height and go face first, it should work. Put yourself out of this misery."

I stepped back from the railing, my hands shaking and my eyes welling with tears. I could picture the scene perfectly. I could see myself tipping over the railing, falling headfirst like an Olympic diver into a pool. I could feel the force of gravity yanking me to the pavement below.

I could hear the final thought I would have right before impact: "Why me?" Then, like an angel hovering over my lifeless body, I could see myself flopped out across the cement, my skull cracked, my face flattened, my brains splattered everywhere.

I fell back through the already open door to my apartment and curled into a ball, sobbing on the floor next to my couch. I cried for what felt like an hour. Every time I thought I was finished, another wave of deep emptiness and sadness would hit me, and tears would flow down my face. My abs hurt and my head pounded. I didn't care anymore if my two other roommates walked in and saw me bawling on the ground. I didn't care about much anymore. I was broken.

I was petrified of my own mind, but not because I had had a suicidal thought. Those types of thoughts had become familiar, they happened often, and I always met them with a stern "no" and my will to live. Tonight was different, though. I was worn out. I was exhausted from constantly battling my brain. I was scared my life would be like this forever. Now, for the first time, I had softened to the idea that suicide might be a viable option. I just wanted to stop suffering. If the rest of my life was going to be like this, then why continue living? I revisited this question over and over in my head that night.

I couldn't understand how I'd wound up this way. I'd grown up with a loving mother, father, and sister in Indianapolis. All things considered, my childhood was great. I went to a good school, played sports, and hung out with my friends. When I graduated from high school, I moved an hour north to attend Purdue University. While there, I rushed and pledged Sigma Chi and studied business. College went by way too fast. After graduating, I packed a U-Haul full of what little belongings I had and moved to Raleigh, North Carolina, to start my career working for the technology company Cisco Systems.

I was a part of their early-in-career sales program comprised of thirty to forty kids my age. Every day we learned about Cisco's technology and how to get really good at selling it. After work, we would all get together and hang out. Everything was great . . . for the first year.

Then, seemingly out of nowhere, as winter set in, I started waking up with what felt like a drumline in my chest. My palms would be sweaty, my mouth would be dry, and my mind would be racing. I had no idea what was going on, but I knew I didn't like it. I decided to keep what was happening to me to myself and try to figure it out on my own. In all of my infinite wisdom, I determined that my brain had flipped a switch, like how someone turns a lamp on and off, and all I needed to do was flip it back to the way it had been before.

I resolved that I would accomplish this by spending January "cleaning" myself up. I'd rid my body of toxins by working out every day, relaxing in the steam room at the gym, and avoiding alcohol and marijuana. I'd stay in on the weekends, rather than going out and socializing. So that's what I did—every single day—for thirty-one days.

And I did get results—just not the results I was looking for.

By the end of the month, not only had my symptoms of anxiety intensified, but I also felt guilty, sad, and worthless. That was depression. If you're experiencing that right now, you know how scary it can feel. Like a thick, gray fog rolling over the hill and into my life, it completely sucked the beauty out of everything around me. My senses had been dulled, and my legs felt like bricks.

I was twenty-three years old, living in a new city far from home and battling a foe no one else could see and that I couldn't understand.

This went on for months, and I got really good at doing two things: hiding what was happening from the people around me, and denying what was going on in my mind even to myself. I told myself I just needed more sleep. I just needed to stop partying so hard and drinking too much. I just needed to stop smoking pot. I just needed to work out more. I just needed a vacation.

As the days passed slowly and painfully, my anxiety morphed into full-blown panic. A voice in my head started to tell me that nobody at work liked me. It would tell me that I was worthless and that I didn't deserve my job. It would tell me that I wasn't likeable. I would ruminate over every conversation I had with friends and people at work. "Did I sound stupid?" I would wonder, and the voice would respond, "Of course you sounded stupid. It's *you* we're talking about, isn't it?" This voice would tell me I wasn't good-looking, that I was terrible at things I enjoyed, and that I was a failure.

Then things took an even darker turn. The voice inside my head started to tell me to kill myself. At first this thought would only come into my mind once or twice a day. I would do my best to ignore it. I might've been suffering and miserable internally, but I wanted to live. I loved life! But I started thinking about it more and more frequently. Now, it would start from the moment I woke up to get ready for work. "Just kill yourself," my brain would tell me. "You're already miserable, so why not?"

Within months of the onset of these symptoms, I was thinking about ending my own life from the moment I opened my eyes until my head hit the pillow at night. I thought about it while driving in rush-hour traffic to work, sitting at my desk, making phone calls, conducting performance reviews, eating lunch, working out at the gym, heading home from work, sitting on the couch with my roommates, and right before I went to bed. Sometimes I would even dream about it. No matter where I went or what I did, the overwhelming dread and desperation were always there.

By this point, I was crying a lot, late at night in my room by myself, so my two other roommates wouldn't hear me. The next morning, I would drag myself out of bed, get dressed for work, and head into the office, always making sure to paint on my mask of false exuberance and competence. I didn't want anybody to know me as Zach the Weak, the guy who couldn't figure it out. But my energy to battle these feelings and fake it to the outside world was fading. I was tired of fighting my own brain. I was tired of pretending everything was okay. Life didn't seem worth living anymore.

That April was when I found myself on the floor of my apartment sobbing after picturing myself going headfirst off the balcony. I knew that if I didn't do something different, I would probably end up taking my own life. Through racing and confused thoughts, I decided there was one last thing I could do. I would call my parents and let them know how severe things had gotten. During our previous conversations, I'd described some of the symptoms I was dealing with, but I always tried to pretend like things weren't that bad. Tonight was different. I felt like I was fighting for my life.

Choked up and with tears in my eyes, but still trying to act casual, I told my parents about the suicidal thoughts I was having. I told them how miserable I felt every single day and how hopeless I felt about my future. I told them I couldn't go on much longer feeling like this. Words and tears poured out of me. Once I finished, there was a pause on the other end of the phone.

My parents told me, "Zach, we think it's time you go seek help."

I could tell they were very concerned but didn't know exactly what I needed. They just knew that I had to seek medical attention as soon as possible. I had never considered this as an option. My whole life I'd thought going to a psychologist meant you were either crazy or weak. Strong people didn't need to go to a shrink. Strong people figured things out on their own. I didn't want to be considered crazy or weak. I wanted to figure all of this out by myself.

Now, on the darkest night of my life, the people I had always wanted to be proud of me were telling me it was okay to get help. As we hung up, I promised them I would take the time to try and find someone who could help me.

The very next day, I started to make phone calls around town to schedule an appointment. I wanted relief, and I wanted it fast. After a bit of trial and error, I eventually found a psychologist who understood what was going on with me. In late 2016, nearly a year into this arduous journey, I was diagnosed with an anxiety disorder known as obsessive-compulsive disorder (OCD) and started a talk therapy wellness plan. I utilized exposure and response prevention (ERP) to treat my symptoms. And it started to work.

The Road to Recovery

The decision to get professional assistance from a qualified doctor is a major reason why I am who I am today: a much more content, happy, and healthy person, who has learned to cope with anxiety and depression. However, my road to recovery has not been easy, and it's taken time. Through my journey I learned how important it is not to try and figure out everything on your own, but instead to have help every step of the way. I built my team, and I also acquired some tools outside of professional treatment to support my recovery. I want to share these tools with you, so that you, too, can decrease your feelings of anxiety and depression and live a more fulfilled life.

You picked up this book because you don't want to continue at college or in the first years of your professional life feeling the way you feel. First, congratulations! Realizing recovery is possible is a huge step. Second, I want you to know that I'll be there with you every step of the way, and together we'll create your brain health blueprint (more on this terminology in a bit). I'll be your guide, walking hand-in-hand with you, as you start to put together the pieces to this puzzle, in order to start feeling better and get the most out of this time in your life.

To be clear, I am not a clinical psychologist, therapist, or doctor. My unique understanding and skill in this area comes from my personal experience reclaiming my own life. In the process, I learned a lot about building a brain health blueprint that supports positive mental health. These days, in my work as an advocate and speaker, I travel to colleges around the country. I talk to people who are going through what you're going through all the time, and I coach them through their challenges.

My goal is to provide you with hope, through my story, that recovery is possible and to help you understand that you are not alone. There are millions of people around the world who are coping with and building better mental health for themselves every single day. My hope is that, by learning more about how your brain works, you'll start to treat yourself a little better and ultimately realize your fullest potential.

Let's Smash the Stigma

Throughout this book, you'll see me refer to mental health as *brain health*. I do this in part to help undo some of the stigma associated with the term *mental health* and because the brain is an organ, and it's within our power to take good care of it, just like we do our other organs. Consider that we don't refer to heart health as *soul health*. Our heart is tangible, and we can take steps to protect and strengthen it. Heart disease and other heart illnesses are challenges that people face, but it's culturally understood that we should take care of our heart's health to manage and prevent such challenges. The same is true for our brains. Although our brains are the most complex organ in our bodies and there is much to learn about them, we are capable of taking specific, research-supported steps to improve how they function. Brain health, therefore should be looked at as an important part of our lives and something we take care of. For the purpose of this book, you can think about brain disorders, brain illnesses, and brain issues as the challenges we potentially face with anxiety, depression, or the onset of more serious psychiatric illnesses such as schizophrenia or OCD. I am not trying to rewrite how the healthcare industry refers to our mental health. Rather, I am encouraging you to think about our brains in a slightly different manner. As a tangible object that can be cared for just like our hearts.

THE BRAIN IS AN ORGAN, AND IT'S WITHIN OUR POWER TO TAKE GOOD CARE OF IT, JUST LIKE WE DO OUR OTHER ORGANS.

PART 1

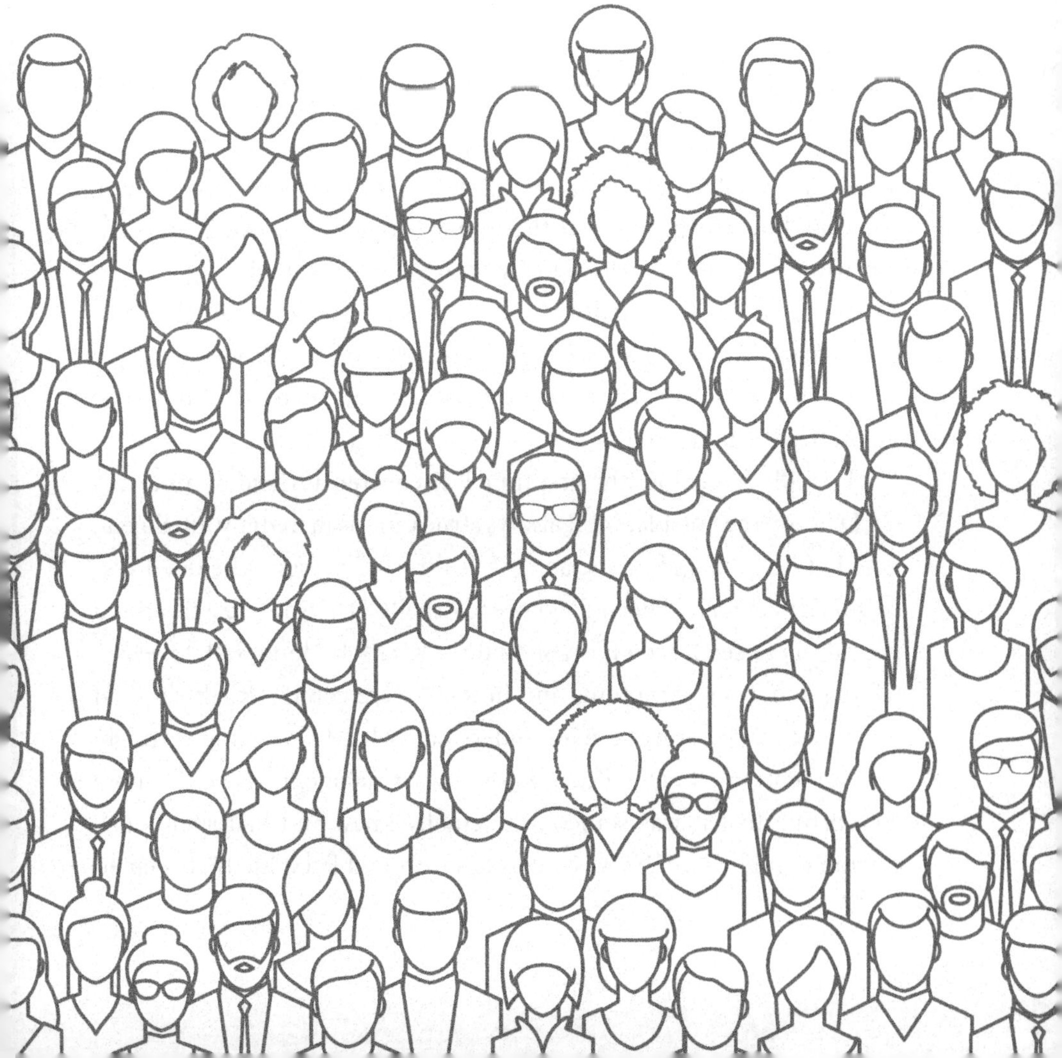

CHAPTER 1

YOU ARE NOT ALONE

You might be thinking you're the only one in your friend group struggling with anxiety and depression. You might even feel like you're the only one on the face of the planet dealing with these challenges. These beliefs can, understandably, make you feel pretty isolated. After all, how frustrating is it that other people get to live a "normal" life, while here you are dealing with your symptoms solo?

But consider that plenty of people around you are struggling just like you are. You just can't see it, because, like you might, lots of people keep it to themselves. The way someone presents themselves in public might be very different than how they actually feel.

I vividly remember the first time I discovered a friend of mine had OCD. From the outside, she'd always struck me as incredibly intelligent, gifted at her job, ambitious, and a self-directed person. The day I discovered she, too, had been diagnosed with OCD, it was like a thousand pounds had been lifted off my shoulders. We took a long walk together, talking about our symptoms and how we were coping. It felt so good to connect with someone who understood what I was going through, not to mention a huge relief to know I wasn't alone. It was even more comforting that it was someone I actually knew and had spent considerable time with. She was a good person and led a life that seemed well-balanced. For the first time in nearly half a year, my feelings of isolation and hopelessness were replaced by hope.

It took me way too long to learn that lesson, which is why I'm sharing that story with you now. The reality is that you are not alone. Not even close. There are literally millions of perfectly sane, high-performing, "normal" individuals who live with anxiety and depression all over the world.

I believe there are three groups of people living in the world today. The first group are those people who are currently living or dealing with some type of brain health issue like anxiety or depression. The second group are those who will experience some type of brain health issue in their lifetime. The third group is those who will know someone living or dealing with a brain health issue. So, through that lens, it's safe to say that we are *all* affected by brain health, and therefore we need to learn how to empathize with and support each other through our struggles.

WE ARE ALL AFFECTED BY BRAIN HEALTH, AND THEREFORE WE NEED TO LEARN HOW TO EMPATHIZE WITH AND SUPPORT EACH OTHER THROUGH OUR STRUGGLES.

The Numbers Don't Lie

The likelihood that you know someone coping with a brain health challenge like anxiety, depression, or suicidal thoughts is high. According to the 2018 *State of Mental Health In America* report published by Mental Health America, 43 million American adults have a brain health condition like anxiety or depression. That's enough people to fill the University of Michigan's football stadium, the largest in America, almost four hundred times! Nearly half of those with a brain health condition have a co-occurring substance abuse disorder. Nearly 21 million American adults experience suicidal ideation, and 57 percent of American adults with a brain illness have not received treatment. The Anxiety and Depression Association of America (ADAA) reports that anxiety disorders are the most common brain illness in the US today. According to the organization's report, anxiety disorders affect 40 million adults over the age of eighteen. The ADAA says that nearly 75 percent of those affected by an anxiety disorder will experience their first episode before the age of twenty-two. It is estimated that 50 percent of Americans will experience some type of brain issue like anxiety or depression in their lifetime.

When looking at college students specifically, the numbers are equally astounding. According to brain health research conducted by the National Alliance on Mental Illness, one in four students has a diagnosable brain illness. Of those students dealing with a brain issue like anxiety or depression, 40 percent of those surveyed didn't seek the treatment they needed. A 2018 study conducted by the American College Health Association revealed that, in a twelve-month period, 55 percent of students reported feeling things were hopeless; 88 percent of students reported feeling overwhelmed by all they had to do; 84 percent reported feeling exhausted (not from physical activity); 42 percent reported feeling so depressed it was difficult to function; and 50 percent had become so anxious they struggled in school, making anxiety the most common student brain health problem on campus.

Depression is the number one reason students drop out of school. If it's left untreated, it can lead to other symptoms—or worse. Suicide is the second leading cause of death among college students, claiming the lives of eleven hundred students each year. More than half of college students have had suicidal thoughts; 67 percent tell a friend they are feeling suicidal before telling anyone else; and 13 percent have seriously considered suicide in the last year. The vast majority who die by suicide were not receiving help from their college counseling centers.

Young adults also report being lonelier than their older counterparts. A nationwide survey conducted by health insurer Cigna discovered that more than 50 percent of respondents felt alone or left out always or sometimes. People scoring 43 and above were considered lonely in the survey, with a higher score suggesting a greater degree of loneliness and social isolation. The younger generations, Gen Z and

Millennials specifically, scored the highest on the survey. Members of Generation Z, those born between the mid-1990s and the early 2000s, had an overall loneliness score of 48.3. Millennials, just a little bit older, scored 45.3. By comparison, Baby Boomers scored 42.4. The Greatest Generation had a score of 38.6 on the loneliness scale. Simply stated, younger generations feel lonelier and more isolated, which is contributing to brain health challenges.

Keep This in Mind

You don't need to feel like an outsider or loner any longer. That belief is only going to bring you down and make you feel worse about yourself. And it's simply not true. No matter what you're going through right now, I guarantee you there's someone close to you who is also suffering in silence. I've traveled all over the country speaking to hundreds of students, sharing my personal story and smashing the stigma around anxiety and depression. Time after time, students will approach me afterward to share their personal struggles. Each story is powerful and reminds me that we are not alone.

CHAPTER 2

YOU ARE NOT GOING CRAZY

When feelings of anxiety kick in, it's not uncommon to believe you might be losing your mind. In part, that's because the thoughts that stem from anxiety can feel so persistent, distressing, and urgent. You may not understand them or know where they're coming from, which can lead to these thoughts feeling all the more intense and even compounding on each other.

One of the first steps in getting a handle on anxiety is recognizing it when it's occurring. Of course, being worried or fearful from time to time is human, and is not necessarily indicative that you're dealing with anxiety. If, for example, the town where your family lives is anticipating a hurricane or blizzard, it's natural to be concerned for their well-being. It's when your worries and fears persist and intensify in a way that becomes disruptive to your life that you might want to take a closer look at where they're coming from and see if you can notice a pattern. Using the example above, you might begin to realize you are dealing with anxious thinking when the hurricane or blizzard has long passed and your brain is coming up with new ways to fear for the safety of your family. You might find yourself constantly checking in with them to make sure they're okay, which interferes with your ability to do your schoolwork.

Here are a few examples of fears and/or worries you may or may not identify with anxiety:

- Worrying that you'll get stuck in a situation or place you can't get out of or leave when you want
- Fearing something terrible will happen to yourself, a friend, or a family member
- Worrying that you've forgotten to do something important, like turn off the stove or lock the door
- Stressing that something needs to be done perfectly
- Wondering if someone you care about is upset with you as you wait for a text back from them
- Feeling unsure if you look stupid in a social setting
- Convincing yourself you have that rare disease like cancer
- Believing nobody likes you
- Fearing that you will fail miserably at something
- Having intrusive violent thoughts like you'll suddenly snap and harm someone
- Having intrusive sexual thoughts like questioning your sexual orientation
- Feeling anxious about being anxious
- Referring to the list above, another example of when anxiety could be manifesting itself is obsessing and ruminating over a social interaction you had with your roommates. You might worry and debate in your head for hours at a time over whether or not you said or did the right thing in front of them. This might lead to you obsessively debating whether they like you.

Vicious Thinking

All of these thoughts are, of course, valid and common. The issue is that people with anxiety tend to get caught in what I call the "vicious thinking vortex." The "vicious thinking vortex" is the tornado-like funnel people like myself, and you, can spiral down when experiencing anxious thinking. At the top of the funnel is the hole we can fall into that starts the whole process of worrying. You might have a thought like, "I wonder if I really like girls?" This thought is normal, and many college students explore their sexual orientation. You consider yourself a heterosexual male, though, so when you have one of these thoughts, you might think, "Why did I have that thought? Could this thought be true?" An individual without anxiety might have a thought like this and be able to shrug it off as something random. However, if you're dealing with anxiety, you might be more susceptible to the vicious thinking vortex, when that thought pops up in your head and you begin to ruminate and experience feelings of stress or anxiety. You might think, "If I had this thought, then it *must* be true. How can I really be sure though? What if I'm actually gay?! I can't stop this thinking or this feeling. I must be going crazy!"

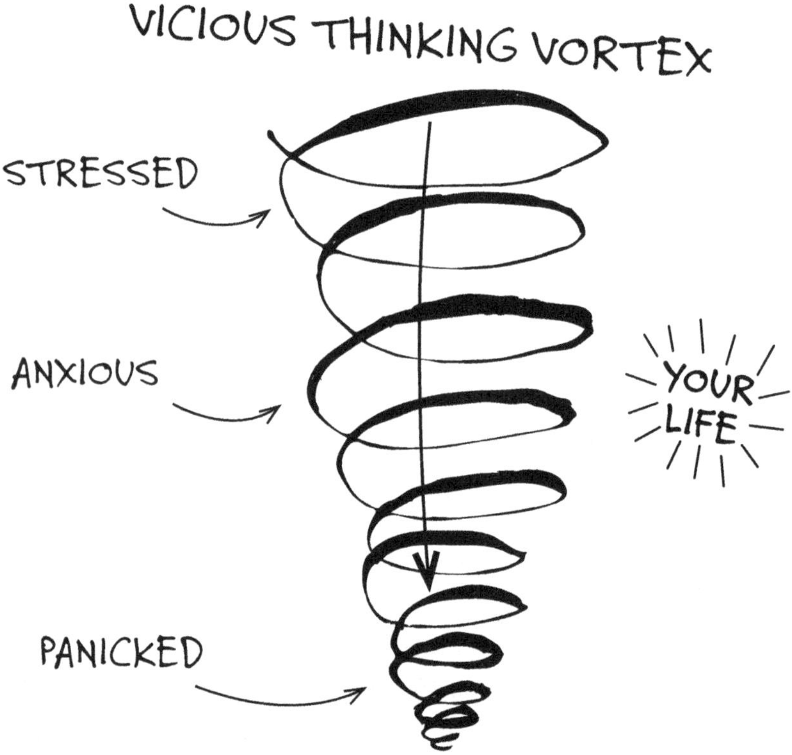

As you give more and more weight to these thought patterns, you begin feeding your anxiety by ruminating on the original thought. This spikes your anxiety levels even more, which sends you further down the vortex. At the peak of really intense anxiety, you find yourself at the bottom of the vortex, where you feel extremely overwhelmed, like your head is spinning. In some cases, this intense anxiety can lead to a panic attack, which is the sudden intense feeling of terror without a threat of actual danger. Furthermore, if you convince yourself you're going crazy, or you feel like the thoughts you're having are in conflict with who you are, this can cause feelings of lower self-worth, which can lead to feelings of depression. This one question or thought has now completely consumed your thoughts. It's important to know this is a completely normal reaction for people with anxiety and you're not alone.

When I first started experiencing anxiety, I remember thinking, "Whatever is happening to me right now is not me. It's not how normal people's brains work. I just want my brain to go back to how it was before. I'm going to keep this to myself and figure it out on my own." I did everything I could to distance myself from what was happening in my mind. I wanted to hide what was going on internally from the people around me. I didn't want people to know I was dealing with a brain health issue because I thought it was weird. I was ashamed of the thoughts I was experiencing, I didn't know why I was having them, and I didn't have a clue who to turn to. I kept telling myself, "This isn't me. I am not a crazy person. I am not weak, and I can fix this on my own. I am not one of *those* people." I ended up convincing myself I had gone crazy, because no matter how hard I tried to suppress them, the thoughts only got worse.

All of this may hit close to home for you. Your next question might be "But why is this happening to me?" The truth is, our brain's core function is to keep us alive. We naturally approach certain aspects of our lives with doubt and fear because that helps us make smart decisions that ensure our survival. For people like you and me, who may struggle with anxiety and depression, our brain's negativity bias can be turned up a bit more and be more persistent. For example, someone without a tendency toward anxious thinking might have a thought about having cancer, be frightened, but brush off that thought and move on with their day. Someone like you and me might have a similar thought, feel fear and anxiety, and then ruminate on that thought for days, weeks, or even years looking for evidence that we indeed do not have cancer. In this example, two people have the same thought, but one person is able to shrug off the thought and move on, while the other will have increased feelings of anxiety even after getting confirmation that they don't have cancer.

If you've ever been stuck in the vortex of vicious thinking, you're not going crazy and you're not losing your mind. Instead, you're experiencing a reaction that's totally normal for people with anxiety. Your anxiety causes fears and worries to *feel* more real and creates a tendency to believe them. I've had all the thoughts and experiences listed above, and over time, I've learned to change my relationship with them, which has significantly reduced my anxiety (more on that later). What's important for you to know right now is that the more you buy into your thoughts (ruminating on them, looking for evidence of them, etc.), the more anxiety you will feel, and the more they will consume your day-to-day. This will inevitably cause you higher levels of anxiety, and cause you to think you are going crazy. When in reality you are a bright, beautiful, outstanding human being with all the potential in the world to do great things.

THE MORE YOU BUY INTO YOUR THOUGHTS, THE MORE ANXIETY YOU WILL FEEL.

CHAPTER 3

YOU ARE YOUR BIGGEST ALLY

You might feel embarrassed or guilty about your feelings of anxiety and depression. Maybe you think, "What do I have to be sad for? I have a great life. There are people who have it way worse than I do. I'm fortunate to be going to this school and to have friends who care about me." Maybe you've been to a party recently with friends you love, and though cognitively you understand that you should feel joy, you don't really feel anything.

In other instances, you feel ashamed of how you feel: "Why can't I just feel happy? Is there something wrong with me? Am I just not a strong enough person to get over my issues?" You feel like you don't deserve to feel the way that you do, and it's got you stuck in this vicious cycle of thinking poorly about yourself. Maybe your grades aren't where you want them to be, and you feel like a failure. I feel your struggle because I've been there, too.

I didn't seek professional help for so long because I was ashamed of what I was feeling. When my depression really started to sink in, my internal dialogue constantly beat me up. I would make myself feel guilty for feeling depressed. Sometimes my thoughts would just go off on me: "Why do you have to feel this way, man? Literally, your life is fine! You're lucky to have the job that you have. You have friends to hang out with all the time. Hell, you even have a new girlfriend. Plus, your friend who just lost her sister. She's allowed to be sad, not you. There are people in this country and around the world living in poverty right now that don't even know where their next meal is coming from, and you have the audacity to feel depressed!" I let this dialogue rule my thinking until I didn't feel like living anymore.

You need to understand that you don't need to justify your pain. It's just as valid as the next person's. You are allowed to feel however you feel, no matter what. It's okay to not be okay. Period. Everybody's struggle is unique to them. You don't need to have lost your mother in an accident, lived in the poorest neighborhood, and been abused as a child to feel like your feelings of depression are acceptable. Of course, those factors, which we will discuss in more depth later in the book, can contribute to feelings of depression, but they're not requirements for your depression to be okay. You feel how you feel, and that's that.

IT'S OKAY TO NOT BE OKAY. PERIOD.

If you're struggling academically, socially, or for any other reason while at school because you're coping with feelings of anxiety or depression, you need to communicate with your parents and the school. Don't look at the challenges you're dealing with as an excuse and as a result suffer in silence. Clinical depression and anxiety are both medical conditions that warrant the same level of respect as any physical challenge.

Think about this: if you were struggling in school with your grades because you had been diagnosed with cancer, would you look at having cancer as an excuse? More than likely, you wouldn't. You would look at it as a valid reason for why your grades aren't great. So why don't you see your brain health challenges in the same way?

Another example I like to use is with runners. Let's say you were a great marathon runner, the same way I know you're a great student, or else you wouldn't be in college. One day you're running along, and you roll your ankle so badly you sprain it. What would you do? Would you hide your sprained ankle from everybody and attempt to run 26.2 miles? More than likely, you wouldn't. You would tell someone you were struggling with your ankle. But let's say you did decide to run. Would you be as fast as you were before the sprain? Would you be able to perform at your peak? My guess is no. Well, this is the same for your brain health. Waking up and struggling with untreated depression or anxiety every day while trying to perform at school is a lot like being a marathon runner trying to run a marathon with an untreated sprained ankle. Your performance simply won't be as good until you address the issue by working with medical professionals to get better.

Never let somebody else determine for you whether or not you're allowed to feel *any* type of emotion. If a family member, friend, colleague, or anyone else belittles the emotions you are feeling, be aware that they are participating in shaming and guilting. They may not be bad people, generally speaking, but this is an unhealthy and ill-informed approach to helping you cope with what you're feeling. If you choose to buy in to their perspective, this will only make your feelings of depression and anxiety worse. This is because you will start to resist or deny these emotions. Resistance or denial only leaves more space for these emotions to linger, get worse, and intensify. Furthermore, their approach may have the unintended effect of discouraging you from wanting to seek help from a medical professional that can aid in your recovery.

You need to become your biggest ally. Your recovery depends on you rooting for yourself. You have to want to see yourself get better and know that you deserve it. This begins by consciously becoming aware of when your brain starts shaming you and making you feel guilty. For example, your brain might think, "You are really a screw-up. You never get anything right. You must not be strong enough to get over this feeling." Note these thoughts by saying, "I recognize that my brain is trying to make me feel guilty for what I am feeling right now." Then replace that shaming thought with something reassuring and purposeful. You could say, "I might be feeling this way now, but that's not something I need to be embarrassed or ashamed of. I deserve to recover and feel happy."

This isn't forced positive thinking, by the way. This is truth. You don't need to feel ashamed and you do deserve to recover, the same way someone with cancer wouldn't be embarrassed and deserves to recover.

If a friend you love deeply came to you and said they were feeling really depressed and anxious and felt ashamed about it, how would you speak to them? Would you put them down? Would you make them feel even worse than they already do? I'm willing to guess that you wouldn't. You'd want to be there for them and reassure them that they shouldn't feel ashamed or guilty. You would talk to them kindly and supportively. Thinking about things from this perspective makes it so much easier to want to become your biggest ally. Treat yourself the way you would treat a friend who was struggling.

When you become your biggest ally, you open the door to a whole new mentality. You start to look at yourself as a brave warrior who's in control of your brain health. You shed those old, debilitating beliefs that you're weak or cowardly and replace them with the realization that you are strong and resilient. You battle something every single day that nobody else can see, and yet here you are: still living, breathing, and doing your very best. And guess what? That's something to feel really, really proud of.

CHAPTER 4

TAKE BACK CONTROL OF YOUR LIFE

To take back control of your life, you need to know—and believe—that recovery from what you're going through is possible. You can improve your feelings of anxiety and depression and in some cases completely eliminate them. This might be tough to believe at first. You might believe that you're going to feel the way you do forever and that your life is ruined. I once had that belief, too. I thought, "Well, now that my brain has made this switch, these deep feelings of depression and intense feelings of anxiety are just going to be my miserable reality. Every day is going to be a struggle for me, and that's that."

This is because I believed that my brain health was fixed. In other words, I was either mentally well or mentally ill. If I was mentally well, then my life was going to be great. I'd be able to do all the things that make up a successful and happy life: maintain positive relationships, pursue a career path, do things I enjoy, stay physically fit, go on vacations, get married, have kids, and maintain a positive frame of mind. Conversely, if I was mentally ill, well then, that meant my life would be drastically different from other people's. I'd never live a "normal" life again, and the same opportunities wouldn't be available for me.

What I've learned is that our brain health is much more of a continuum that we will fluctuate back and forth on based on different factors in our lives: our genetics, the significant life events we go through, traumas, and daily stressors. All of these factors impact our mood and how our brains feel and function.

Yes, having a brain disorder can be disruptive to your life, but it's not a life sentence. You are more than capable of living a happy, healthy, and productive life no matter what you are experiencing with your brain right now. By understanding the factors that impact your brain health, we'll collaborate to put together the proper brain health blueprint that promotes feelings of well-being and contentment for you.

HAVING A BRAIN DISORDER CAN BE DISRUPTIVE TO YOUR LIFE, BUT IT'S NOT A LIFE SENTENCE.

Factors That Affect Brain Health

Everyday challenges: On a daily basis, there are things that cause you stress, anxiety, frustration, anger, sadness, and doubt. It could be dealing with a tough professor you don't get along with. Or learning to adjust to an early morning class. Maybe you have a roommate who isn't very nice to you, and now you have to figure out how to cope with your living situation. These are just a few examples, but it's critical that you understand that these everyday challenges can drastically impact how you feel and function.

Stress: There's good stress and bad stress. Good stress can be used as a motivator to push you forward and take on the day. This type of stress builds resiliency and mental stamina over time. Bad stress is when you've put way too many things on your daily and weekly agenda, which causes you to feel worn out and overwhelmed. This type of stress leads to irritability, anger, nervousness, lack of energy, lack of focus, and feeling as though you could cry.

According to the American Institute of Stress, 73 percent of people reported having stress that impacted their mental health. The top causes of stress identified in the US were job pressure, money, health, relationships, poor nutrition, media overload, and sleep deprivation. You more than likely feel stress in at least one of these categories. You might stress about getting good grades so you can find the perfect job and make enough money to live a good life. So you work long hours, going to class and studying late into the night. On top of a full course load, you pack your schedule with leadership roles and clubs, and still find time to develop friendships. All of these pressures you put on yourself can cause negative stress and impact your brain health. Can you think of an area in your life that is causing you negative stress?

Lack of sleep: Quality sleep is necessary for your brain to function at peak levels. Adults need seven or more hours of sleep per night to maintain a positive mood and focus. According to WebMD, a lack of sleep has a number of consequences. For starters, sleepiness and sleep deprivation cause accidents. Sleep deprivation was a major factor in some of the biggest disasters in recent history: the 1979 nuclear accident at Three Mile Island and the massive Exxon Valdez oil spill that killed thousands of animals, to name a few. Sleep loss disrupts your thinking and decision-making. This impairs your ability to pay attention, be alert, concentrate, and problem-solve.

Losing sleep can make you gain weight. There is a link between lack of sleep and an increase in hunger and appetite. According to a 2004 study, people who sleep less than six hours a day are almost 30 percent more likely to become obese than those who slept seven to nine hours.

A lack of sleep can also contribute to the symptoms of depression. In a 2005 Sleep in America poll, people who were diagnosed with depression or anxiety were more likely to sleep less than six hours at night. Insomnia, the most common sleep disorder, has the strongest link to depression. How many hours of sleep do you get a night?

Low self-esteem: In psychology, the term *self-esteem* is described as a person's overall sense of self-respect or personal value. In simple terms, it describes how much you appreciate and like yourself. Self-esteem can involve a variety of beliefs about yourself, how you feel about the way you look, your capabilities, your emotions, and your behaviors. Too little self-esteem can leave you feeling like you don't have much to offer or contribute. It also can cause you to feel low levels of self-respect.

Low self-esteem can lead to unhealthy choices, like enduring abuse in a destructive relationship or not living up to your full potential because you don't believe in yourself. This is why self-esteem is important and plays a significant role in your mood, motivation, and outlook in life. Low self-esteem may hold you back from taking on new challenges at school because you don't believe you're capable of success. On the flip side, a healthy self-esteem can help you achieve because you're able to navigate the highs and lows of life with a positive outlook and assertive attitude, and you believe you'll accomplish your goals.

Signs of healthy self-esteem:

- Confidence in your abilities
- The ability to say no
- A positive outlook on life
- The ability to see overall strengths and weaknesses and accept them
- An overall perspective that's not impacted by negative experiences
- The ability to express your needs
- An understanding that past failures don't define you or your capabilities
- Feeling grounded in your beliefs

Signs of low self-esteem:

- A negative outlook on life in general
- Lacking confidence in your abilities
- An inability to express your needs
- A focus on your weaknesses
- Believing that others are better than you (inferiority)
- Trouble accepting positive feedback
- A fear of failure

Environmental: These factors can include verbal, physical, or sexual abuse. If you have been the victim of any type of abuse, it's important to know that it has potential to impact your brain health. It can cause feelings of lower self-worth, lower self-esteem, guilt, shame, fear, anger, and sadness. These are completely appropriate reactions to a traumatic event like this. If you're the victim of any abuses I want you to know that you deserve justice, recovery, and happiness. You can find the National Domestic Violence Hotline in the back under the resources section.

Financial: Financial instability can be one of the biggest factors in your day-to-day brain health. You might feel pressure to perform in school because your parents are paying for some or all of it, and therefore they have high expectations. You could be a first-generation student whose parents used a good portion of their savings on your tuition. Maybe you're on scholarship. Or perhaps you constantly worry about whether you'll have enough money to pay for your books, classes, meals, and rent. All of these scenarios can cause you to experience chronic stress. If this stress builds up over time, it can create additional health complications, like feelings of anxiety or depression.

Burnout: Another factor that can impact your brain health and increase feelings of stress, anxiety, and depression is work burnout. According to the Mayo Clinic, job burnout is a state of physical or emotional exhaustion. From my experience, this can be caused by feeling constant pressure to succeed at work, working long hours, or conflicts that arise with your boss or colleagues. Signs of burnout might include fatigue; using food, drugs, or alcohol to feel better; disrupted sleeping habits; unexplained headaches; or increased feelings of anxiety or depression.

Race: To you, the person of color reading my book now, I want to first recognize that as a white male in America, my experience of growing up has been different than yours in some ways. Primarily, I have never felt the trauma and pain of being discriminated against because of the color of my skin. It breaks my heart, and I will do everything in my power as a white male to recruit my white brothers and sisters to be actively antiracist so we can make this country truly equal, so you feel safe and comfortable to seek professional help.

That being said, as a person of color you may have experienced race-related traumas that cause feelings of chronic stress, anxiety, and depression. On top of these traumas, you might feel hesitant to seek help for culturally based reasons, fear of judgment, and a belief that the psychologist won't understand you because of cultural differences. You might feel uncomfortable opening up to a white professional because you're worried they won't understand struggles that are specific to you. For that reason, I have provided a list of resources at the back of the book, like TherapyForBlackMen.org, so that you feel comfortable, understood, and safe opening up to a therapist. I am with you every step of the way to support you on your journey to healing and happiness.

Traumatic life events: According to Healthline, a traumatic event is an incident that causes physical, emotional, spiritual, or psychological harm. The person experiencing the distressing event may feel threatened, anxious, angry, sad, or frightened as a result. Traumatic events include, but are not limited to, the death of a loved one, divorce, a breakup, a major illness, an accident or injuries, war, natural disasters, or job loss. All of these events have the potential to impact your brain health in the short and long-term. For that reason, it's important that you address these challenges by engaging in the recovery process.

Transitions: A transition is a major change—as in moving into a dorm and being away from your parents for the first time, or changing your major. Transitions will be a never-ending process for the duration of your life, and they can be scary. I will never forget my transition from high school to college. I hugged my parents goodbye and watched them drive away. I thought to myself, "Wow, I'm really on my own now." I was excited to be gaining this independence, but also fearful. I had no idea what to expect. I wasn't certain I would be able to make it in college.

You might be feeling the same way because a transition has occurred in your collegiate career. Just remember that change can cause feelings of uncertainty, which has an impact on your brain health. When you're going through a transition, you might do things you otherwise wouldn't do because you want to fit in. You might feel lost because there is no clear next step. These feelings are completely normal, and I promise you, you are not weird for feeling them.

Mental health disorders, developmental disabilities, and genetics: Scientists and doctors have known for a long time that all major psychiatric disorders have a heritable component. In other words, the genes you receive from your parents do influence whether or not you will develop a brain disorder. For example, anxiety disorders like OCD and major depressive disorder are inherited 20–45 percent of the time. Bipolar disorder, schizophrenia, ADHD, and autism spectrum disorders are closer to 75 percent inherited. Scientists are investigating which genes drastically increase the likelihood that you'll develop a psychiatric disorder and how that process unfolds. Talk with your family to better understand what brain health challenges have impacted your relatives. Once you know your risk factors, you can consult a doctor to understand how to properly take care of yourself, the same way you would if there was a history of cancer or heart disease in your family.

The Continuum

The factors above can and will impact your brain health and your experience on the brain health continuum. Once we realize all the factors in our life that can impact our brain health, we see that maintaining positive brain health is a balancing act that requires daily attention. If you look at the following image, you will see the five core areas on the spectrum: **Balanced Life, Difficult to Balance, Needs Assistance to Balance, Needs Constant Assistance to Balance, and Not Able to Balance.** It's important to remember that figuring out where you are on this continuum at any given time is not intended as a means to judge yourself, but rather to provide an honest evaluation so you can recognize if and when you need assistance.

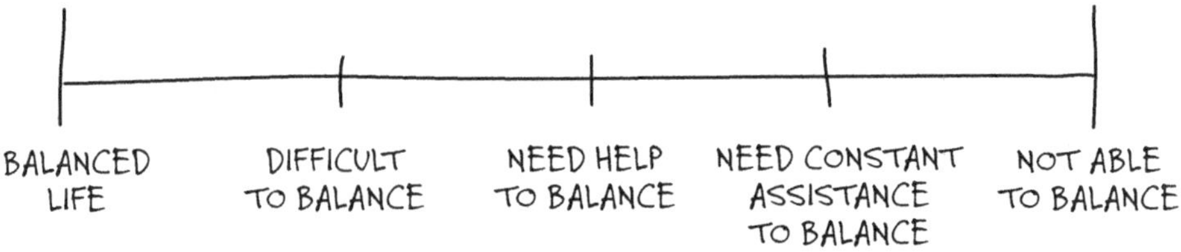

Balanced Life: In this state, you are consistently content and have a satisfied mind. You have a positive outlook, focus on good habits like getting enough sleep and exercising, and have healthy strategies to lower stress levels. You maintain relationships that are positive and mutually beneficial for your brain health. In this state, you are able to realize your full potential, can cope with the normal stresses of life, can work productively and fruitfully, and are able to make a contribution to your community. Keep in mind, this does not mean there is an absence of a brain disorder. It means that you are effectively managing your disorder while maintaining a balanced life.

Difficult to Balance: In this state, you are content and satisfied most of the time but could be dealing with factors that are affecting your outlook on life. Perhaps you have a really tough class and you dread the very thought of attending it because you don't like the professor or the curriculum. You might have a packed schedule that consumes a lot of your energy. These factors might cause additional levels of stress or frustration that make it challenging to balance a positive brain state. However, once the semester is over, and you finish the class, you are able to regulate your emotions and maintain a feeling of positive life balance. Keep in mind, this does not mean there is an absence of a brain disorder. It means that you are effectively managing your disorder while maintaining a balanced life.

Needs Help to Balance: In this state, being content and satisfied is more challenging and requires some outside assistance. Maybe you have just experienced a significant event in your life, like a breakup. As a result, you are experiencing depression and learning strategies to cope with these feelings of rejection and loss. Since these feelings are new to you,

you are seeing a therapist and leaning on your close friends to help you through this tough time.

In this state, your outlook on life could be less positive. It's important to remember, though, that we all have times in our lives where we need to lean on others more than usual to get through. Over time we can migrate back to a balanced life. Keep in mind, this does not mean there is an absence of a brain disorder. It means that you are effectively managing your disorder while learning to cope with other factors and maintain a balanced life.

Needs Constant Assistance to Balance: In this state, maintaining contentment and satisfaction requires regular outside assistance. Perhaps you've been diagnosed with obsessive-compulsive disorder and are really struggling to cope with the symptoms. You are learning methods to help maintain positive brain health, but for now you need regular assistance from a psychologist, a peer support specialist, and your family and friends. At this spot on the continuum, it's important to remember that you aren't necessarily going to be here forever. With a commitment to recovery, regular treatment, medication, coping strategies, and support from your social circle, you can slide closer to the balanced life side of the continuum.

Not Able to Balance: In this state, it's not possible to be content and satisfied. You might have just received news about the death of a loved one. You might've been diagnosed with a severe brain disorder. As a result of this death or diagnosis, you are in a very dark place that makes it extremely challenging to lead a normal life. In this state, you might isolate yourself from others or spend large portions of the day in your room or lying on the couch. Your eating and sleeping patterns may change. It might be difficult to just get up and shower.

As a result, you might not be able to go to class and might need to take time off. Being in this state does not make you weak or helpless. It means you are human and struggling with a very tough time in your life. At this place on the continuum, it's important to remember that what you're going through isn't necessarily permanent. It will require that you seek professional medical assistance to help express your emotions and learn coping strategies. You might need to move in with family or close friends to have a regular support system close by. This is completely fine and encouraged. You are having a human response to a very traumatic experience. Not being able to balance your emotions now doesn't mean this will be the case forever. With proper medical and social support, you will eventually begin to edge your way closer and closer to living a balanced life again.

If you're at a less than optimal place along the brain health continuum right now, there's always the possibility your life can be more balanced. Building out a brain health blueprint that will be effective for you takes intention and commitment, but bouncing back from anxiety and depression *is* possible, and you'll be all the more resilient for having had this very human experience. If you don't already, by the end of this book, you're going to feel confident that you can take control of your life and own your brain health.

You are very close to feeling a lot better. Keep pushing. Let's do this.

PART

2

CHAPTER 5

UNMASKING ANXIETY AND DEPRESSION

Your brain is not broken. You are not going crazy. I say this not to make you feel better, but because it's true. Instead, you are having normal reactions to feelings of depression and anxiety that are caused by the many factors we discussed in the previous chapter. However, the symptoms that come with anxiety and depression can be scary and distressing to the person experiencing them. They can feel like they hold control over you. But by understanding and normalizing the symptoms of anxiety and depression, you'll be able to take away some of their power. Let's take a closer look at what these symptoms actually feel like and the different bodily sensations that accompany them.

The Nuts and Bolts of Anxiety

The root of anxiety stems from a complex set of brain structures known as the limbic system, also referred to as the "emotional brain." In 1915, physiologist Walter Cannon coined the term "fight or flight" specifically about this part of the brain. The core function of this system is to perceive threats and then keep you alive by either avoiding or confronting those threats. You probably know what it feels like when this system is at work in your body, like right before you're about to give a speech. You feel your heart beating rapidly as adrenaline rushes through your body. Or when a friend jumps out and scares you. You get a jolt through the body that focuses you, and your palms become sweaty as you react instinctively. The fight-or-flight response happens in a split second. This is great because it helps us react quickly and keeps us alive!

What makes the limbic system unique for people dealing with anxiety, though, is that it doesn't seem to want to shut off. Our brains jump from one worried thought to the next, even when there isn't a real threat. This can cause a lot of distress and all sorts of reactions in the body. These reactions can cause us to fear our bodily sensations, which can feed more anxiety. Therefore, it's important to understand what those responses are, so we're not surprised or caught off guard by them. Let's look at some of those different bodily sensations now.

Pounding heart with chest pain: When I first started to experience anxiety, it felt like I had a drumline in my chest. I would wake up and my heart would be pounding for no apparent reason. My lungs would feel tight, and pain would shoot through my chest down my arm. I felt like I had just sprinted away from a lion, but since I couldn't point to anything obvious, my brain invented the idea that I was having a heart attack. This is one of the most common concerns for people with anxiety. Many people end up in the ER because they think they're on the verge of a heart attack, when in reality they're experiencing a symptom of anxiety. (Do tell your doctor if you have any concerns about heart health or underlying cardiac conditions.)

Shortness of breath: At times you might feel like you can't catch your breath, which might cause panic and fear to kick in. You might think, "What will happen if I can't breathe properly in a public place?" or "What if I'm unable to catch my breath and need to go to the hospital?" Like pouring gasoline on a fire, when you buy into these anxious thoughts, your shortness of breath may intensify. Because of the way you're breathing, there is a slight drop in oxygen and blood supply to the brain, which can lead to dizziness and confusion. You might fear that you'll faint.

Feeling on edge: This is that added layer of tension you feel throughout your body, like when you've been sitting down too long and become fidgety. This feeling of edginess is the result of nervous energy created in the body when you feel anxious. Think of it like a bouncing ball stuck inside a metal box, ricocheting from one wall to another, looking for an escape. The buildup of this anxious energy can cause discomfort in your body, making you feel like you could scream or punch something as a way to release to it.

Muscle tension: You might notice a lot of tightness in your neck, upper back, and shoulder muscles. This is caused by your fight-or-flight response, which prepares you for action by tightening those muscles. When you experience anxiety and stress on a regular basis, tension builds in those muscles, causing you to feel tight and stiff.

Twitches and tremors: When nervous energy builds up in the body, you might sometimes feel muscle tremors or twitching. You might experience this in your chest, arms, or legs. For me, I know I've let anxiety and stress build up too much without releasing it when my eyelid starts to twitch.

Sweating: This is an automatic response triggered during fight or flight as the body works to cool you down. When you are experiencing anxiety, you might notice you have sweaty palms or dampness under your arms. Although it might not be the ideal reaction, know that this is a sign your body's natural response is working.

Dry mouth: Your mouth can feel completely void of saliva when anxiety kicks in. This can make it difficult to swallow or talk. This feeling can cause discomfort and make your throat feel dry as well.

Stomach pain and nausea: When you feel butterflies in your stomach, this is actually the fight-or-flight response moving blood from your digestive system to your muscles and other vital organs. The challenge with this is that it can cause pain or the feeling that you might throw up. This can increase anxiety because you might fear vomiting in a public area and embarrassing yourself in front of other people.

Dizziness and tingling: Anxiety can cause tingling sensations throughout your body. (I once leaned over to a friend during a movie and asked him to make sure I didn't die if I had a heart attack because I could feel tingling in my fingers. Of course, this was simply a common reaction to anxiety and something I didn't need to fuel with more fearful thoughts.) In addition, you might feel dizziness. This is caused by increased respiration. When you're anxious, you tend to breathe too rapidly (hyperventilation), which causes that feeling of lightheadedness. You might believe that you'll faint. Although possible, it's extremely rare because your blood pressure goes up when experiencing anxiety, and fainting is caused by low blood pressure.

Worry and derealization: You might find yourself constantly worrying as your brain plays scenarios over and over again in your head. This is because your limbic system is on high alert. It is vigilant in preparing you for perceived threats that may or may not be real. Maybe you recognize that the fear and worry you can't let go of is silly, so you argue with your brain, going in circles about this threat. Eventually your worry about these threats becomes a worry about your thoughts, and you begin to fear the contents of your mind. The fear of going crazy, potentially harming someone, or being sick starts to feel very real.

A less discussed sensation is derealization. This occurs with individuals who have been struggling with anxiety for an extended period of time. It's a sense of unreality, as if the world you're living in isn't real. You might question your very existence or feel like you're in dream. Health Research Funding reports that up to 66 percent of people who experience a trauma will have some form of derealization. Although scary, it's important to know it's actually one of the most common symptoms of anxiety.

Mind going blank: As anxiety increases, your mind can go blank. For me, this happens all the time. Even as a public speaker, I still experience high anxiety before speaking, and on some occasions my mind goes blank. This is a very normal side effect of anxiety.

Avoiding situations, people, and places: You might have noticed that your anxious thoughts have caused you to entirely avoid certain situations, people or places. This is because you believe that, by avoiding the situation, person, or place you fear, nothing bad will happen. You also believe that, by avoiding the situation, person, or place, you won't trigger the thoughts that cause you to feel fearful and anxious. For example, you might fear that by going to the party your friend invited you to, you'll do something extremely embarrassing and everyone will judge you. You might fear losing control and causing a loved one physical harm, so you avoid situations or objects you fear could do that. Avoidance is a normal behavior for people with anxiety and something you should be aware of so you can respond accordingly. (We will discuss this in the next chapter.)

The Mechanics of Depression

Just like anxiety, everyone experiences feelings of sadness, loneliness, or grief during difficult times in their lives (remember the continuum). You might feel sad because of a breakup. Maybe you feel down because you studied really hard for a test and didn't get back the grade you expected. You might be feeling blue because you just had a falling-out with a friend. These feelings of sadness, loneliness, or grief are all part of the human experience. You're supposed to feel these emotions, even if we don't always want to. In most cases, when you feel these emotions, they go away after a short period of time, and you're able to bounce back to normal everyday life.

However, what happens if those feelings of sadness linger or become excessive? What if your sadness is keeping you from completing schoolwork, disrupting your sleep, or making it difficult to enjoy activities you once loved? What if you're feeling fatigued or worthless?

Depression is a medical condition that goes beyond life's ordinary ups and downs. People with depression cannot simply "pull themselves together" and get better. When someone is experiencing symptoms of depression, daily life becomes a chore. Simply getting out of bed in the morning could feel like the biggest task. Treatment with counseling, medication, or a combination of both are keys to recovery.

DEPRESSION IS A MEDICAL CONDITION THAT GOES BEYOND LIFE'S ORDINARY UPS AND DOWNS.

Extreme sadness: When you're depressed, you feel deep sadness. This isn't the type of sadness that comes and goes relatively quickly. Instead, this feeling tends to creep into your life slowly and intensifies over time. It might feel like your whole world has been washed over in gray. Things that once brought you joy and happiness no longer do. You might be in situations where you know you should feel happy and still feel nothing but sadness. This is the most common feeling, and it can be scary, but you can get better.

Feeling emptiness: I remember once standing on the beach in Lake Tahoe, looking out at the crystal-blue lake surrounded by beautiful mountains and feeling the warm, yellow sun shining down on my face. As I stood there, I tensed every muscle in my body and focused intently on trying to conjure up feelings of happiness. I wanted desperately to feel something, but all I felt was numbness. I felt empty and completely void of emotion. I knew I should be happy in this situation, but I couldn't change how I felt. You might be feeling this exact same way. It's not a great feeling in the moment, but I promise you it won't last forever if you take action.

Feeling like you could always cry: If you're experiencing crying spells often, this could be a sign that you're feeling depressed. Frankly, I always felt on the verge of tears. I used to sit in my apartment alone, staring at a blank TV, and would just start bawling. Whether or not you're prone to crying, if you notice an uptick in the amount of crying you're doing, then this could be a sign you need to seek professional assistance.

Withdrawal from others: One of the most typical behaviors depressed people exhibit is isolation. For whatever reason, when you're depressed you just don't want to be around people or have to talk to them. You might notice you're isolating yourself more often in your room and not coming out for entire days. You might spend entire days or weeks in your bed and not want to interact with friends or family.

Weight loss or gain: You may not have an appetite, or the thought of food might be nauseating. On the other hand, you might be eating a lot more than usual. As a result, you might have gained or lost weight in the last few months. I lost about twelve pounds at the peak of my depression because I couldn't eat. No matter what I did, I simply didn't have an appetite.

Sleeping too much or too little: For some people, feeling depressed causes them to sleep all day. They just want to escape from what they're feeling, so they sleep. You might be experiencing the same thing. Maybe you really struggle to get out of bed in the morning or are sleeping in until the afternoon. Maybe you can't sleep at all. You might find yourself tossing and turning all night long. You stare up at the ceiling, hoping that you'll fall asleep, but it never happens.

Fatigue: According to a 2018 report, fatigue affects over 90 percent of people with major depressive disorder. You might be feeling tired, too. You wake up and your brain is in a fog. Your eyes are bloodshot and dry, and you have no energy. This feeling lasts for days, with little to no improvement. This is potentially caused by sleep issues, diet, stress, and even the medications used to treat depression.

Feelings of guilt: As we discussed earlier, it's very common for people coping with depression and anxiety to feel guilty. You might've noticed yourself feeling like you don't deserve to feel sad. Maybe you don't want to feel like a burden to other people. Whatever the reason, if you're feeling guilty, just know this is a sign of depression and not something you need to buy in to. You're allowed to feel how you feel, and that's that.

Reoccurring thoughts of death or suicide: You may be having thoughts of suicide or death. Maybe you've envisioned driving yourself off the side of the road. Or maybe you've pictured yourself dead and daydreamed about how people would respond to that. This is a very common side effect of depressed thinking. For reasons not totally known, depressed individuals idealize suicide and death. For me, when my depression was at its worst, I thought about suicide from the moment I woke up until the moment I went to bed.

If you are experiencing thoughts of suicide, it's critical to know thoughts of suicide do *not* need to be acted on. When your brain is in a depressed state, it's a great liar. It tries to tell you suicide is a viable option. It attempts to convince you that you'll feel this way forever, so what's the point in existing? This simply isn't true. Once you've healed your brain and those symptoms of depression have subsided, you'll see with a clear mind that you want to live and your brain was lying to you.

If you're reading this right now and feel like you need immediate help, reach out to the National Suicide Prevention Lifeline at 1-800-273-TALK or the Crisis Text Line by texting TALK to 741741.

Body Health vs. Brain Health

Just like your brain health, your physical health is a continuum as well. Think about a time in your life when you felt like you were in peak shape. During this time, your physical health was dialed in. You felt strong, confident, and proud of how you physically felt and looked. You probably were nourishing your body with the proper nutrients. Maybe you were going to the gym and accomplishing important benchmarks toward your ultimate fitness goals.

However, let's say one day you woke up with the flu, and because you were feeling run down, you weren't able to make it to the gym. Since you were sick, your body felt weak. As a result, you were unable to make it to the gym for a few days. Would you say you were in peak physical shape then? Probably not, because you were sick and your body was recovering, and as a result you shifted on your physical health continuum. Ideally, you relaxed and rested up, binged on a few Netflix shows, and got the medicine you needed to get back on track.

In that example, something as simple as coming down with an illness altered your physical state of well-being. This caused you to slide over a bit on the continuum to a place where you needed a little bit of assistance to get through the next week or two. You probably went to the MinuteClinic or your campus doctor to get a checkup and figure out what was going on, so you could return to a balanced state. In this case, we've been conditioned to seek help for common physical illnesses.

Now, imagine that you're going on a run down a path you had never run on before. As you're running, your foot slips into a pothole and you twist your ankle terribly. Immediately, nerves in your legs shoot signals to your brain indicating you have pain in your ankle. Before you know it, your ankle is swollen to the size of a baseball, and you can't move it at all. As you limp along the trail back to your car, you realize you can't put any pressure on it whatsoever. You manage to get back to your car, drive back to your place, and collapse onto the couch. You are so ashamed of your physical injury that you decide you're going to hide it from your roommate, your sibling, and your parents. You don't want them to ever know that you hurt yourself, so you decide you're going to live the rest of your life hobbling around. You don't want to seek medical assistance for fear of judgment.

Does the end of this scenario sound right to you?

No, it doesn't! After severely injuring your ankle, you would more than likely call your roommate for help and head to intensive care to get your ankle looked at. You would tell your parents. The doctor would provide you with a recovery plan, and over time your ankle would heal. You might need assistance from others to carry your books so you could use crutches. No one would judge you or look at you as weak or weird. They would want you to recover so you could get back to normal life activities. So why is it so different with our brain health? Why do we resist seeking treatment when something feels off with our brain balance? It's because of the way we've been conditioned to look at physical health compared to brain health.

Studies show that people have more empathy around physical injuries and illness than they do with brain challenges. However, when we compare brain health to physical health, we realize that both are continuums and very common. What we learn from this example is that both brain health and physical health deserve equal respect and attention. Our brain and body health are interconnected, and therefore both need to be cared for.

When you have an issue with your body, you go to a doctor, receive a diagnosis, and get put on a treatment plan. When you have an issue with your brain health, you go to a qualified doctor, receive a diagnosis, and get put on a treatment plan. It truly is that simple. And why wouldn't you want to get help for your brain? It's the most important organ we have and the one that differentiates us from every other living organism on the face of the planet.

When Should You Get Assistance?

Take a second to revisit the symptoms for anxiety and depression. If you have three or more of these symptoms for most or all of the day, nearly every day, for at least two weeks, and the symptoms are intense enough that they're interfering with your daily activities, you may be experiencing depression, anxiety, or both.

If that's the case, it's time to get some help, and fortunately you have lots of options. We'll look into them in the next chapter. For now, the most important thing to remember is that all of these symptoms are treatable. I repeat: *all of these symptoms are very treatable.* Please do not make a permanent decision based off of temporary emotions. You might not feel like yourself right now, but I promise that with treatment and patience your symptoms can drastically improve and you can begin to live a happy and fulfilling life.

CHAPTER 6

KNOW YOUR TREATMENT OPTIONS

There are many different forms of treatment that when administered properly can effectively improve your symptoms of depression and anxiety. These can include talk therapy, medication, or a combination of both. Since I'm not a licensed professional or doctor, I'll talk about these approaches based on my personal experiences, as well as the extensive research I've done on effective treatments. It's important to face your brain health challenges head on by seeking the right professional assistance. After all, running away from your problems only increases the distance between you and the solution. The easiest way to escape the challenge you're facing is to run toward it and solve it.

Cognitive Behavioral Therapy (CBT)

What is it: CBT has been proven in clinical trials to effectively treat depression, anxiety, panic attacks, schizophrenia, sleep problems, eating disorders, and some of the other life stressors we discussed earlier. In this therapeutic and practical approach, a therapist works with you to examine how your thoughts about certain situations have the potential to impact the way that you feel and behave. Your therapist focuses on the present day and how challenges are affecting you in your life now. Working with your therapist, you come up with goals that help you more effectively cope with these challenges.

As an example, you might be invited by friends to attend a fraternity party. This invite causes you to start thinking negative thoughts. You might feel anxious and scared. You might become worried that you'll do something embarrassing or that people at the party won't like you. As a result, you may decline the invite, avoiding your friends completely, or you go but use alcohol or drugs to cope with the situation.

Here's another example: Maybe you get a poor grade on an exam. This grade might cause you to think negative thoughts. This causes you to feel frustrated, angry, and sad because you don't feel like you're smart enough or good at anything. Because of these feelings, you might act out by snapping at friends and family members, or you might start to think studying is pointless because you'll never get better grades.

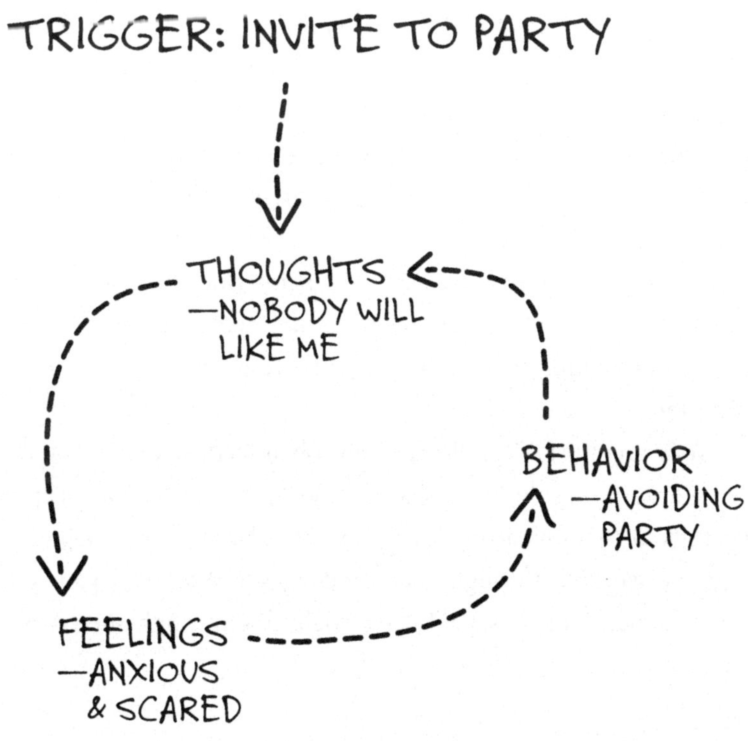

Over time, these cycles of thoughts, feelings, and behaviors start to become habitual. You start avoiding situations more and more, or you automatically start blaming yourself for "perceived failures." The more you reinforce this vicious cycle, the worse it can get. You can become stuck in this pattern of thinking.

A CBT therapist will help you break this cycle by figuring out what types of negative feelings, thoughts, and behaviors could be contributing to the challenges you are experiencing. They'll help you examine your negative thought patterns and change your behavior.

What to expect: If you're picturing yourself lying down on a couch while a bearded man in glasses interprets your dreams and examines every detail of your past, think again. When working with a CBT therapist, you should expect a very practical approach that focuses on present-day challenges and goals to improve outcomes. Although you might look into past thoughts and behaviors, it won't be the focal point of your sessions.

This process is extremely collaborative. It's really meant to be a team approach to examining the issues you're struggling with, where your psychologist and you work through your challenges together. You can expect to get assignments to work on between sessions, to practice the skills and the strategies you learn in-session out in the real world. Just like physical therapy, if you do the assignments outside of your therapy sessions, odds are you'll make progress and improve at a much faster rate.

Your therapist will welcome and solicit feedback from you on how things are coming along. This is great because it creates a team approach where your therapist is not an authoritative figure but somebody who's with you working through your challenges and refining your goals to improve your outcomes. CBT can be delivered through one-on-one sessions, in groups, via self-help books, or online.

Acceptance and Commitment Therapy (ACT)

What is it: This therapy is grounded in the belief that all humans have a need to control their thoughts and feelings. For example, you might want to get rid of your feelings of depression, anxiety, fear, anger, grief, and so on. Through your internal struggle to eliminate these thoughts and feelings, you create more suffering for yourself as you battle back and forth with them.

In ACT, there is no attempt to try and reduce, change, avoid, suppress, or control these emotions. Instead, ACT teaches you to reduce the impact and influence these unwanted thoughts and feelings have on you through the use of self-acceptance, mindfulness, commitment, and behavior-change strategies to help you create a rich and meaningful life. It aims to help you embrace your thoughts and feelings rather than fight or feel guilty for feeling them. In turn, this therapy steers you into taking effective action, which is guided by your deepest values while working to be fully present and engaged. Although the goal of this therapy isn't to reduce anxiety or depression, what research has shown is that individuals who participate in this type of therapy do experience lower levels of anxiety and depression as a byproduct of the treatment.

How it works: There are six core principles of ACT.

- Cognitive defusion
- Acceptance
- Contact with the present moment
- The observing self
- Values
- Committed action

Cognitive defusion: This is the process of learning to perceive your thoughts, images, memories, and other cognitions as nothing more than bits of language and words that bubble up. They are not what they appear to be—threatening events, rules that must be obeyed, and objective truths or facts. This process helps you to neutralize thoughts and feelings that cause you discomfort.

Acceptance: In this phase of ACT, you learn how to make room for unpleasant feelings, sensations, urges, and other internal experiences. Through this process of acceptance, you allow these experiences to come and go without holding onto them, struggling with them, trying to avoid them, or giving them weight. From my personal experience, developing the skill of acceptance is one of the biggest reasons I don't experience debilitating anxiety like I used to. I no longer allow my thoughts to hold power over me. I genuinely don't care whether or not I have certain thoughts or feelings. Instead, I let them float by like clouds in the sky.

Contact with the present moment: You might find your mind racing with thoughts that create internal dialogue you can't turn off. Don't try to turn these thoughts off because it will only cause more turmoil. Instead begin to develop the skill of cultivating awareness of the here and now. This skill set can be difficult to build at first because you might feel like you're swimming upstream against the current of negative thoughts. Rather than looking at this as an aggressive process of forcing yourself to swim upstream to get to the present-moment "destination," imagine yourself floating on an inner tube that moves with the current, as you gently focus on the activity you are doing on the inner tube. You are not trying to remove the stream below you, but instead you accept its existence while simultaneously engaging in whatever you are doing.

The observing self: This is the process of beginning to understand that you are not your thoughts, feelings, memories, urges, sensations, roles, or even your physical body. Instead, you can view yourself as an outside observer of your own thoughts and understand your thoughts and feelings as transient or impermanent. By developing the skill of outside observation, you create a layer of separation between your thoughts and how you identify with them. You no longer have to believe every stream of thoughts or feelings that bubbles up in your mind, but instead recognize that thoughts and feelings come and go just like clouds in the sky.

Values: In this phase, you clarify what's most important to you, deep in your heart. You become clear on what type of person you want to be, the life you want to live, and what's meaningful to you. This could mean identifying that you value building meaningful friendships, helping other people, and spending time with family. You can use your values as the force that creates willingness to feel unpleasant emotions like anxiety or depression and still participate in activities you enjoy. For example, you might be willing to feel anxiety in a social setting in order to create the opportunity to develop a meaningful friendship—something you value.

Committed action: Now it's time to set goals based on your values and then take effective action to achieve them. Using the example above, this could be setting the goal to attend an earth science class social gathering, to make one new friend who's interested in the same things as you. You'd be able to do this knowing that no matter how you feel, you are not your thoughts or feelings, and you can accomplish what you value through committed action.

What to expect: An ACT-trained therapist will be an empathic listener and an active guide during your therapy sessions. During these sessions, you can expect your therapist to encourage deeper exploration and nonjudgmental awareness. Sessions might include mindfulness exercises that help you develop the skill of healthy awareness of thoughts, feelings, sensations, and memories that you've otherwise avoided. Through this process, your therapist will use cognitive exercises to help you rewrite old narratives and then align new actions you can take to get you closer to your personal values. ACT therapists may assign homework to practice in between sessions, like mindfulness exercises. All assignments outside of therapy will be agreed upon between you and your therapist in advance.

Exposure and Response Prevention (ERP)

What is it: If you've been diagnosed with OCD or believe you might have OCD, then ERP is the most effective form of treatment. ERP involves exposure to a feared stimuli and the simultaneous prevention of rituals that are performed because of the anxiety-provoking stimuli. These stimuli could be unwanted thoughts, feelings, images, objects, and situations. The key to this form of therapy is to confront your anxiety and obsessions while also making a commitment to not give in and engage in compulsive behavior. Through this process of exposing yourself to feared stimuli and then preventing physical or mental compulsions, you begin to habituate to these thoughts and feelings. Over time this will cause a drop in anxiety levels.

Here's an example: Let's say you have recurring thoughts that you are going to cause physical harm to someone you love. When you have these thoughts, your fight-or-flight response is activated and you feel high levels of anxiety. To avoid triggering the thoughts of actually harming someone, you avoid being in situations where that person will be there. You might also avoid touching or picking up objects you believe could harm someone, like a kitchen knife, out of fear that you might snap and actually do something. You then ritualize by reassuring yourself that you would never do something like that. This is in an attempt to reduce your anxiety and rid yourself of these thoughts.

How it works: Using the example above, you would engage in exposure and response prevention with a licensed mental health care professional who specializes in ERP. Next, you would participate in a series of in-person sessions where you would deliberately expose yourself to the thoughts that cause you anxiety and fear. These exposures would be done in a systematic, phased way to ensure that you're not putting too much on your plate at once, which might cause you to quit treatment. Over time, you and your therapist would work together to habituate you to the intrusive thoughts you're having. Through this process, you can significantly improve feelings of anxiety and depression and reduce the frequency of intrusive thoughts.

Common obsessive feelings and thoughts:

- Fear of being contaminated by germs
- Fear of losing control and harming yourself or others
- Intrusive sexually explicit or violent thoughts and images
- Excessive focus on religious or moral ideas
- Fear of losing or not having things you might need
- Focusing on order and symmetry; the idea that everything must line up "just right"

Medication

Since I'm not a qualified doctor who prescribes medication for a living, I won't be providing guidance in this area. What you should know is that taking medication for a brain health challenge is not something you should be ashamed or embarrassed of. If you are considering taking medication to help with your feelings of anxiety and depression, make sure to consult a doctor and do some research on the side effects of the medication being recommended to you.

For a lot of people, medication is refined through trial and error. This means you might need to work closely with your psychiatrist early on to figure out what type and dosage works best for you. Another thing to consider is that different psychiatrists specialize in different brain health challenges. For example, some psychiatrists know how to more effectively treat OCD with medication, while another doctor might be more familiar with treating clinical depression.

Above are a few of the most effective talk therapies to help treat anxiety and depression. This list is not exhaustive, but it should serve as a starting point as you explore ways to improve your symptoms of depression and anxiety.

The key to success for all of these forms of treatment is your willingness to put in the work, the same way you would to rehab a sprained ankle or regain your cardio health after undergoing heart surgery. You get out of therapy what you put into it. More input equals better output. Now it's time to put together the steps to getting treatment, so you can take action and start to recover.

YOU GET OUT OF THERAPY WHAT YOU PUT INTO IT.

CHAPTER 7

HOW TO GET TREATMENT

I sometimes like to think about the process of recovery like an overcast day. You might feel like you've looked out the window for as long as you can remember and it's either been raining or overcast. You might've begun to believe that that's just how the weather is always going to be. However, at some point the sun inevitably begins to break through the dark clouds. Before you know it, it's shining down. You go outside and feel the warmth on your face and body. Eventually the clouds dissipate, and the blue sky that was always there behind the clouds reappears.

How Do I Know If I Need Assistance?

I'm happy you asked! As a rule of thumb, you should always default to seeking professional help. In fact, I believe everybody should have a therapist, since we all have brain health and all face challenges. Whether it's going to see a doctor, therapist, counselor, psychologist, or psychiatrist, getting assistance is always the answer. One of my biggest regrets is not going to seek help the second I started to experience symptoms that were causing me distress. It wasn't until I became conscious that my symptoms were serious and treatable that I realized seeking professional assistance was my best option.

Unfortunately, more than half of all college students have had suicidal thoughts, and yet half of these students have never sought counseling or treatment. Studies show that individuals who seek assistance earliest are far more likely to recover quickly. This is because early care provides you with the medical attention you need to receive a diagnosis, get put on the correct treatment plan, and develop healthy coping mechanisms. This is the same with our physical health, too. The sooner we seek medical attention, the sooner we can begin to heal. To reinforce what we discussed earlier, here are some signs you may want to speak to a brain health professional.

Signs in adults:

- Prolonged feelings of sadness
- Feelings of extreme highs and lows
- Excessive worrying
- Intense feelings of anxiety that occur consistently
- Social withdrawal
- Confused thinking
- Irritability or strong feelings of anger
- Delusions or hallucinations
- Struggling to cope with daily problems and activities
- Substance abuse
- Changes in sleeping and/or eating habits
- Thoughts of suicide
- Excessive complaints of physical ailments
- Racing thoughts or pounding heart
- Feeling like life is pointless
- Constant stress at work
- Repeatedly telling yourself you're a failure
- Irrational fear of failure
- Believing if you weren't alive no one would care

Where to Start

The nature of the issue and/or the symptoms you are experiencing will determine where you go for help. Please remember that finding the right therapist or professional is a process that's unique to you. Don't abandon your efforts if you don't match perfectly with your first medical professional. If I had quit after my first psychologist appointment, I might not be in the position I am today. It took persistence and patience while I sorted through people to find the right fit.

FINDING THE RIGHT THERAPIST OR PROFESSIONAL IS A PROCESS THAT'S UNIQUE TO YOU. DON'T ABANDON YOUR EFFORTS IF YOU DON'T MATCH PERFECTLY WITH YOUR FIRST MEDICAL PROFESSIONAL.

1. Start with a mental health assessment. Start by consulting your doctor, counselor, psychologist, or psychiatrist. The purpose of a mental health assessment is for you and your practitioner to get a better picture of your current thoughts and feelings. These assessments can aid in helping diagnose brain health challenges such as anxiety and depression.

If you're looking to do a quick and free assessment online to get started, check out Mental Health America's (MHA) online assessment or the Substance Abuse and Mental Health Services Administration's (SAMHSA) online screening tools. You can also use other resources like PsychologyToday.com or Psycom.net, which have various assessments. Please keep in mind that these are just preliminary assessments.

Before you take an assessment, take a little time to think about:

- Your current symptoms
- The thoughts, feelings, and behaviors that have been troubling you
- Your family history (Does depression or anxiety run in the family?)
- Has there been a significant event that's brought on these symptoms?
    - A big move across the country

    - Starting a new semester or internship
    - A breakup with your boyfriend or girlfriend
    - Family-related issues
    - Issues with friends or bullying
    - The death of someone close to you
    - Abuse of any kind
- How frequently do you experience these symptoms?
- How long do these symptoms last?
- How are they impacting your current day-to-day life?

Additionally, prepare a list of any prescriptions or other substances you are taking. This is important because some prescription and illicit drugs can impact the way you think, feel, and reason, which might explain some of your symptoms.

2. Understand the different designation of counselors. It's important to understand what your options are. Below is a general list provided by Mental Health America.

Psychologist: A professional with a doctoral degree in psychology who's trained to make diagnoses and provide individual and group therapy.

Psychiatrist: A medical doctor with special training in the diagnosis and treatment of mental and emotional illnesses. Like other doctors, psychiatrists are qualified to prescribe medication.

Clinical Social Worker: A counselor with a master's degree in social work who's trained to make diagnoses and provide individual and group counseling.

Licensed Professional Counselor: A counselor with a master's degree in psychology, counseling, or a related field who's trained to diagnose and provide individual and group counseling.

Mental Health Counselor: A counselor with a master's degree and several years of supervised clinical work experience who's trained to diagnose and provide individual and group counseling.

Certified Alcohol and Drug Abuse Counselor: A counselor with specific clinical training in alcohol and drug abuse who's trained to diagnose and provide individual and group counseling.

Marital and Family Therapist: A professional with a master's degree, with special education and training in marital and family therapy, who's trained to diagnose and provide individual and group counseling.

3. Be prepared when you meet with your therapist or doctor. If you're struggling, it might be difficult to completely articulate how you're feeling or why you're feeling the way that you do. Make sure that you take the time to consider the answers to some basic questions you'll most likely be asked.

- What brings you here?
- Have you ever seen a therapist before?
- What is the problem from your viewpoint?
- What are the symptoms you're experiencing?
- What makes the problem better?
- What is your background?
- What is your life currently like?
- What do you do? (i.e., student, full-time employee)
- Where do you live? Whom do you live with?
- What is your family dynamic like?
- What is your friend situation like?
- What are you looking to get out of these sessions?

4. Start your search for a healthcare professional. Since you're a student on campus, you can always start by scheduling an appointment with your school's health and wellness center. They typically have brain health professionals as well as graduate student staff members who can assist you. That said, over a five-year period campus wellness centers have seen a 40 percent increase in the number of students using their services, so it could take a while—up to six weeks—to land an appointment.

If you can't wait that long (I know I couldn't have), look off campus. Get a referral from your family doctor. If your parents have insurance, their insurance company can provide a list of providers who are in your plan. You can also check healthcare databases for psychologists, psychiatrists, counselors, and therapists in your area. These databases are helpful because they provide additional information such as certifications, accepted insurance providers, and reviews. For starters, try the Anxiety and Depression Association of America (adaa.org), *Psychology Today* (psychologytoday.com), and GoodTherapy (goodtherapy.org). (I've personally used *Psychology Today* as a resource to look up psychologists in my area.)

An important factor to consider here is their specializations. As I learned the hard way, seeing a psychologist who didn't specialize in ERP and OCD only resulted in wasted time and money. However, it wasn't a total waste because it forced me to take a step back and really think about the symptoms I was experiencing. Once I did that, I was able to start correlating the symptoms I was feeling and what I was reading online about the symptoms of OCD. From there, I found a specialist. If you aren't sure which specialist to work with, that's okay. Start by working with your general practitioner to talk through your symptoms. Seek their guidance on who they believe you should work with next.

Factors to consider:

- Read the healthcare provider's reviews and see what other people are saying about them.
- Their biographies will normally give some indication of what methods they use to treat brain health challenges. Make sure you research those methods and have a general understanding of what they entail.
- See if you can feel out their personality from the picture they have displayed, as well as their biography. You want someone you feel you can trust.
- Verify whether they are in-network with your insurance or not before you schedule an appointment.

- Learn how the payment process works.

When you contact a brain health specialist, here are some questions you should ask:

- Are you a licensed psychologist in this state? Is your license active and in good standing?
- Are you currently accepting new clients?
- Can you provide your services both in-person and virtually?
- Where did you get your degree? What type of training or clinical experiences have you had in treating . . . (e.g., mood problems, anxiety, sleep difficulties, depression, etc.)?
- How many years have you been seeing clients?
- What are your areas of expertise?
- What types of treatment do you use? How effective are they in dealing with situations like mine?
- How much do you charge? Do you accept my insurance?
- What is your availability (morning, afternoon, evening, or weekends)? When is the earliest date I can see you?
- Do you tend to see people for longer-term or for shorter-term therapy?

How Do I Pay for Services and Medication?

Financial concerns should not prevent you from getting help. There are options and people available to assist you with your brain health challenges. With that being said, navigating insurance can be intimidating and a little tricky at times.

If you have insurance:

You or your parents' insurance provider may pay for brain health care not covered by your student fees, which could include long-term counseling, emergency room visits, and medication. Insurance policies vary in terms of how much and what type of brain health care they'll pay for. Therefore, it's important that you begin your wellness journey by going to your provider's health plan website. There, you'll be able to see which providers are in-network, the associated costs, and any benefit limitations. Insurance companies are required by law to offer comparable coverage for brain and physical healthcare coverage under the Paul Wellstone and Pete Domenici Mental Health Parity and Addiction Equity Act. This means that insurance providers in both group health plans and the individual market cannot impose annual or lifetime dollar limits on mental health benefits that are less favorable than any such limits imposed on medical/surgical benefits.

Before moving onto campus, call the number on your insurance card and ask:

- Does my insurance policy pay for mental health services in my area? (This is important because many insurance policies cover treatment only in certain areas.)
- What type of mental health services are paid for by my current insurance policy? (For example, office visits, medication, etc.)
- Is there a preferred list of providers I have to choose from? What's the process if I want to see someone out-of-network?
- Is there a limit on the number of covered visits to see a mental health professional? (Insurance policies will often limit how many counseling sessions they'll cover in a year.)
- Will my insurance plan pay for the services I require? If so, how much of the cost will they cover?
- Will I be responsible for a co-pay? Is there a deductible?
- Do I need any approvals or a referral from my general practitioner before the services are provided?

When calling to schedule an appointment, ask the facility where you plan to receive care the following questions:

- Do you accept my insurance?
- Will you bill my insurance company?

- How do you bill for treatment?

In my case, I had to pay the entire bill upfront and then was reimbursed by my insurance company afterward. This process was not streamlined or easy, but it was worth it. I would look at this as an investment in your health and well-being. It will pay off in the long run as you start to feel better.

LOOK AT THIS AS AN INVESTMENT IN YOUR HEALTH AND WELL-BEING.

If you don't have insurance:

When making the decision to invest in your well-being by seeking care, remember that most institutions of higher learning offer free brain health services through their Counseling and Psychological Services Center (CAPS). They will typically offer anywhere between ten and twelve sessions a year.

If insurance is not obtainable, you can seek help at a local social services agency or a federally qualified health center (community-based healthcare centers that are funded by the government). You can do this by googling "community-based mental health services in my area." This should bring up low-cost, affordable options beyond what your school offers. Call the center directly to understand what the process is to receive services if you don't have insurance.

When calling the facility you would like to receive care from, you should always ask if they offer a sliding-scale fee. A sliding-scale fee is when a provider makes arrangements to meet your financial circumstances by adjusting the cost they charge for certain services. If a sliding-scale fee is an option, you might need to bring proof of income, like a tax form for your entire family, to your first appointment. Ask the clinic what, if anything, you need to provide.

I've included some additional resources at the end of the book, like the National Alliance on Mental Illness (NAMI). They have a helpline that offers free help 24/7.

Paying for medication

If you're trying to determine how to pay for medication, talk with the doctor prescribing it for you. They can work with you or direct you to someone who can help determine if a medication assistance program is available to you. Ask your clinician during your visit if a generic brand is available; they're usually less expensive. In addition, ask your pharmacy if they have discount prescription programs. Major retailers like Walgreens may offer discount programs for generic psychiatric medications.

Transparency is key

Once you're in front of a brain health professional, it might be difficult to express the full truth of how you're feeling or why you're struggling. It's important to answer their questions as truthfully and accurately as possible. Some of these questions might make you feel uncomfortable, upset, or angry. Answer honestly anyway. If you're not fully transparent, you might inadvertently create gaps in your treatment plan because your provider won't have all the info they need.

Imagine if you went to a pulmonologist because you were having problems breathing and didn't mention you'd been a smoker for many years. Withholding that information could cause that doctor to misdiagnose you or go down an entirely different treatment path because they wouldn't have all of the information. The same is true for brain health professionals. The more they know, the better they can treat you and get you back on the right path.

Alternative treatment options

Thankfully, with the emergence of online therapy options like Talkspace and BetterHelp, you can now receive therapy from your home, dorm room, apartment, or fraternity or sorority house. Companies like these offer lots of ways to connect, like video, phone, live chat, or messaging. The best part is that you get to choose from thousands of certified counselors across the country. And don't worry about privacy, as you'll be protected by federal HIPAA laws.

If you already have a psychologist you enjoy working with, see if they would be open to doing virtual counseling sessions in the event you cannot come in person. Plenty of mental health care professionals are willing to move their sessions online if that makes connecting easier for you. If you're hesitant about virtual options, you should know that extensive research has shown that virtual therapy can be just as effective as in-person sessions.

Additionally, you can utilize companies like 7 Cups who provide online therapy, as well as support groups. From my personal experience, a support group would have been nice to have when I was in the thick of my symptoms to understand I wasn't alone, weak, or weird. Knowing that other people are going through the same thing as you, gives you the confidence and strength to continue to push forward with treatment so you can get better.

Not discussing the topic won't make it disappear

This is the moment in the book where I put my arm around you and remind you just how important it is that you address the challenges you are facing right now.

"Have you had thoughts of suicide recently?"

It can be hard to believe that someone would ever consider taking their own life. Before I experienced depression, I couldn't fathom suicide. I loved life and everything about it. However, a depressed brain is a brain in pain. If you have been having thoughts of suicide, I want you to know that I've been there, too. It can be a really scary and lonely place. You might feel like nobody understands you or knows what you are going through. Above all else, I want you to know that you are not alone. I am here for you.

CHAPTER 8

THIS TOO SHALL PASS

You might be in a really dark place right now and feel like there isn't much hope left. You might feel like your depression, anxiety, or thoughts of suicide are going to last forever. This makes you feel even lower than you already do because the thought of feeling the way you do for a lifetime seems like too much to handle. You might be thinking, "I didn't sign up for this. My life is not supposed to be this way. If this is how it's going to be moving forward, then I don't know if I really want to live." I understand where you're coming from because I felt that way not too long ago. I once felt like giving up, but my perspective shifted after watching a video that changed my life.

Months after my rock-bottom moment on the balcony, after I'd confided in my parents and been diagnosed with OCD, I found myself still feeling numb, depressed, and anxious. I was happy to have a diagnosis, but I wasn't feeling any better yet.

Shortly after returning from a vacation to Lake Tahoe with my now fiancée, I found myself in my room, tears of frustration and sadness rolling down my face. I had just gone to one of the most beautiful places on the face of the planet and couldn't feel happy. The entire trip I faked a smile but felt agonizing pain secretly. On the plane ride home, I daydreamed about what it would be like if they had brain replacement surgery. I would've been the first one to sign up. I felt that hopeless and trapped.

As I sat in my room frustrated and hopeless, I felt like giving up. What was the point? I decided I would jump on YouTube and watch videos by this guy whose content I enjoyed, Prince Ea. I clicked on the video titled, "I Was Depressed for a Long Time." In the video he talked about how depression was common, so I wasn't alone, which felt good to hear. Then he shared a concept that changed my life.

He said, "I want you to quiet your mind of all these negative and comparing thoughts and just know this too shall pass." He continued, "The biggest thing that depression does is it lies. You feel hopeless, you feel like you don't have any options and you're gonna be in this state forever. Don't fall into the trap of believing that the bad times will last forever. This too shall pass. Never make a permanent decision off of a temporary emotion."

It was a simple video, but I felt a shift in my mood. For the first time in as long as I could remember, I felt hope creeping in. I thought, "I can hold on a little bit longer. I want to see this through to see if these feelings really do pass." I went to my backpack, grabbed a marker and Post-it note, and wrote *warrior* on it. I took that note and posted it by my bedside, so every morning when I woke up I was reminded that if I did my therapy, I could alleviate these feelings. This too shall pass.

Four years later, I have the privilege of letting you know that it's true. Depression, anxiety, and thoughts of suicide really can pass. That's not to say they just magically disappear. You have to put in the work by doing your therapy, living a healthy lifestyle, and taking medication if prescribed. What I am saying is that you no longer have to fear that this is going to be your reality for forever. There is a 100 percent chance that you get through this challenging time if you maintain hope, stay patient, persist, and execute your brain health strategy.

I want you to use this phrase—this too shall pass—as a source of hope. Write it down in your notebook, post it on your wall, and say it to yourself whenever you need a little encouragement. The reality is that energy flows where the mind goes. If you believe you won't get better, you'll never put any energy into trying. However, if you even partially believe

I WANT YOU TO USE THIS PHRASE—THIS TOO SHALL PASS—AS A SOURCE OF HOPE.

that recovery is possible, you'll put energy into your recovery. As you start to make improvements, that belief will become more and more solidified, and you'll get excited about the progress you're making.

The reality is that everything in life is always changing. The *only* constant in life is change. Sometimes you're motivated in school, sometimes you aren't. Sometimes you're in a relationship, sometimes you're single. Sometimes you feel happy, and sometimes you feel sad. Why would it be any different for depression, anxiety, and suicidal thoughts? These emotions you are feeling will pass, and they'll be replaced by new ones. You just have to believe and then take action.

After watching that video four years ago, I still use that phrase today as a source of inspiration and hope because frankly there are still days that suck. Sometimes there are whole weeks that suck. When I'm in one of those ruts, I just remind myself, "This too shall pass. You were in the darkest place of your life not too long ago, and look at you now. This is just another speed bump on the road of life."

No matter what you're going through, do yourself a favor and start believing that this too shall pass. You are not doomed to a life of depression, anxiety, and thoughts of suicide. In time, those rays of sun will break through the clouds and you'll be able to see just how beautiful you and life are. This too shall pass.

Now that you know recovery is possible and that seeking professional help is the best thing you can possibly do for yourself, the next step is to create long-term mindset-based tools to guarantee sustained recovery.

What If I Start to Feel Depressed or Anxious Again?

One concern I hear over and over again from people recovering from depression and anxiety is, "What if these feelings come back? What if I don't stay happy like this and things get dark again?" Maybe you're thinking that, too. The reality is that you might feel these types of emotions again, but you don't need to fear them, because you'll know what it takes to get back on track.

In addition, don't concern yourself with worrying about those feelings on the micro level. What I mean by that is that people who have recovered from depression or anxiety tend to become fearful around if and when they'll start to feel those emotions again. If they start feeling down one day, it might feel like a setback.

As you begin your recovery, try to shift your focus from the micro of your day-to-day happiness to more of a macro focus. Generally speaking, did you feel happy during the week? Overall, did you have a happy month?

This broader thinking will pull you out of the present moment of panic and help you realize that you're doing better than you think. Just because you're having a few down days doesn't mean every day going forward is going to be like that. Instead of believing you're losing control of everything, recognize what's happening and start to work your brain health blueprint to bring your life more into balance. Your brain health blueprint is the set of tools—therapy, mindset tools, and actionable steps (we'll discuss these more a little later on)—you can use to manage your brain health. That might mean meditating more often, scheduling an appointment with your therapist, getting back on your workout routine, or really focusing on getting more sleep. If you drift too far away from the daily steps you take to manage your brain health, that's when depression or anxiety can creep back in.

When you work your plan and stay proactive with your brain health, you'll be more likely to keep yourself in a positive frame of mind and reduce those feelings of depression and anxiety.

PART 3

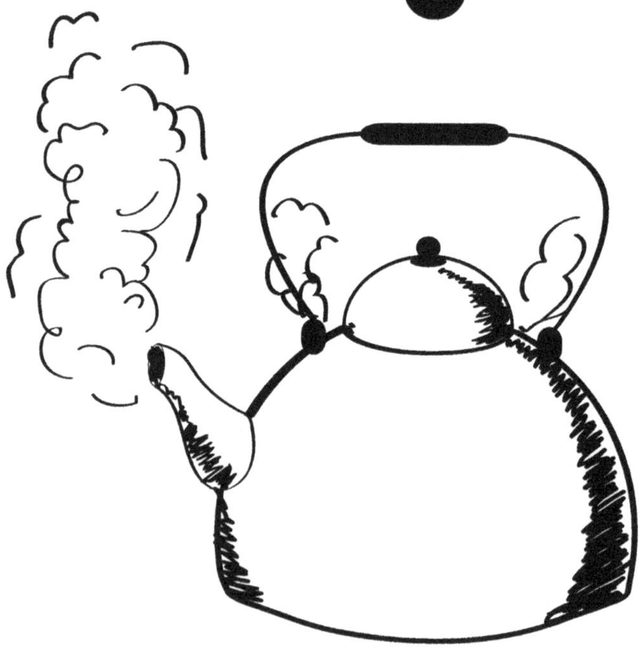

CHAPTER 9

THE TEAKETTLE AND THE STEAM THE TEAKETTLE AND THE STEAM

Imagine a teakettle sitting on a heated stove top. The water in the kettle begins to warm up, so steam starts to build inside the enclosed kettle. As the water gets hotter and hotter, the steam looks for a way to escape. Once the water reaches its boiling point, the built-up steam is forced through a small hole in the spout, and a whistling sound occurs.

Similar to how steam builds up in a teakettle, for people who deal with anxiety and depression, over time, emotions and energy build up in our bodies and brains. When we try to ignore or conceal what we're going through, rather than talk about it, pressure continues to build. Just like the kettle, though, our emotional distress will find a release one way or another. That release could come in the form of an emotional breakdown, chronic fatigue, an outburst of anger, substance abuse, or even a suicide attempt. That's why it's critically important that you share what you're feeling in a constructive way, like in therapy.

There will be tough days, weeks, months, and years. Attempting to push down and deny emotions only gives them opportunities to linger and persist. By discussing your struggles openly with your trusted support group, you release energy from your body. This release of energy helps regulate your mood on a daily basis and allows for you to maintain a balanced life.

Going at It Alone

In late 2017 my fiancée and I moved from North Carolina and New York respectively out to California. I felt like I had my symptoms in a relatively good place. I wasn't feeling depressed or anxious like I'd been at the start of 2016, so I was doing okay. However, as we moved into early 2018, I started to feel the gray clouds of depression rolling back into my life. Internally I started to panic: "I thought I put this behind me. What if this means the depression is back for good?"

Over the next few days, I could feel the depression intensifying. My head started to feel heavy, and it was harder than normal to feel happy. One particular day, my fiancée asked me what was wrong. At first I denied that there were any issues, but she could see in my eyes that I was in pain. So she continued to press, and I continued to deny. Eventually she said, "You know you just need to talk to me. Quit trying to do this on your own and just let me in. How am I supposed to know how you're feeling if you keep it all bottled up? How am I supposed to help if I don't know something is off?"

This gave me permission to feel comfortable sharing my truth, so I spilled my guts. I cried. Then we went on a walk and talked more about how I was feeling. Not only did I feel relief in the moment, but the next day I woke up and my mood had improved. I shared more with her and again woke up the next day feeling even better. Before I knew it, I was feeling like myself again. Just by opening my mouth and telling her that I was struggling, I was able to lessen my feelings of depression. This revelation changed how I felt about sharing my emotions.

Before that turning point, I believed sharing your emotions was a sign of weakness. Especially as a male. Growing up, my dad was not an expressive man, and to this day I've only ever seen him cry once. Additionally, as an athlete I never saw any of my teammates or friends cry or express emotion unless it was anger or frustration because we lost a close game. There were no male role models in my life who openly expressed how they felt. For those reasons, I never developed the skill of expressing emotions without feeling embarrassed or weak.

 The Teakettle and the Steam

Now, I never hesitate to tell the people closest to me when I'm struggling with something. The best part is that it always works. Whenever I let the steam out, I feel relief. As a byproduct, I've also developed deeper relationships because I go beyond the surface level and share more intimate parts of myself. You will also need to develop the skill of opening up in order to maintain long-term recovery.

Vulnerability Is the Key

Vulnerability is a tool you'll need to deploy over the course of your life to achieve long-term recovery. Getting comfortable expressing your emotions will be crucial, and let's face it, being vulnerable can be scary. You might believe that opening up to another person will cause them to perceive you as weak. You might worry that you'll be judged or you'll feel embarrassed because you shared too much. These are understandable concerns, but worries that you'll need to learn to let go of.

Bottling up unpleasant emotions like depression and anxiety only allows them to persist. The problem is that most of us believe vulnerability is a bad thing. We all want to put on a facade that we have everything figured out—even when we don't.

BOTTLING UP UNPLEASANT EMOTIONS LIKE DEPRESSION AND ANXIETY ONLY ALLOWS THEM TO PERSIST.

According to author Brené Brown, a vulnerability expert who wrote the best-selling book *Daring Greatly*, vulnerability causes uncertainty, risk, and emotional exposure. According to her, most of us "spend our lives pushing away and protecting ourselves from feeling vulnerable or being perceived as too emotional. As a result, we often judge when others are less capable or willing to mask feelings, suck it up, and soldier on. Rather than respecting and appreciating the courage and daring behind vulnerability, we let our fear and discomfort become judgment and criticism."

Her extensive research has taught her that our rejection of vulnerability often stems from associating it with dark emotions like fear, shame, grief, sadness, and disappointment—emotions we don't feel comfortable discussing, even though they affect all of our lives. However, vulnerability is also foundational to emotions and experiences we crave, like love, belonging, joy, courage, empathy, and creativity.

Think about it this way: You're vulnerable when you tell someone you like them. You're vulnerable when you stand up for racial equality, mental health, or women's rights. Vulnerability is even at play when you express joy at seeing another friend succeed. You and I would consider all of these essential vulnerabilities in life, and so we teach ourselves to become more comfortable with them. After all, they create opportunities for deeper human connection and growth. Love blooms from vulnerability.

By the same token, there's a lot to gain by being vulnerable about your anxiety and depression. If you want to grow and evolve past these feelings, start by opening up. When you discuss your emotions with people you trust, your body has a chance to release them. The emotions no longer hold power over you because you don't fear them or feel embarrassed. This also opens the door for a deeper relationship with someone, because vulnerability leads to reciprocation. Your friends and family are much more likely to share their struggles with you after you've shared something vulnerable about yourself.

How Much Information Should I Share?

Divulge as much information as you feel comfortable sharing at first. As you build rapport with someone, begin to share more. Finding the right fit with a brain health professional is just like the dating process. You need to feel a connection. You need to feel that this person is listening to you and not just throwing suggestions at

FINDING THE RIGHT FIT WITH A BRAIN HEALTH PROFESSIONAL IS JUST LIKE THE DATING PROCESS. YOU NEED TO FEEL A CONNECTION.

you. My first psychologist wasn't a good fit because of fundamental differences. In her practice, she used religion as a core part of her therapy. When I came to her and told her what I was struggling with, she told me that God and the Devil were waging a war inside my brain. For one, I'm not extremely religious in the traditional sense. I absolutely believe in a higher power, but I'm not fully convinced the Christian God and Devil are all that exist based on all the different religions in the world. Two, I didn't like the idea that a war was being waged inside my brain. I felt like there had to be another answer. It doesn't mean that she was a bad person. It just meant that I needed to find someone who was a better fit and more aligned with my values.

With my second psychologist, I shared much more information about my symptoms, but this didn't happen until after we had built a rapport. She took the time to ask me questions about who I was as a person. When we would meet after a few weeks of not seeing each other, she would pick up right where we left off. She remembered our conversations, which showed me that she cared.

Although divulging personal information with a medical professional is vulnerable and brave and does build trust, it's important to remember that this is their profession. At a fundamental human-to-human level, they do care about your success in recovery, but they're not your new best friend or a parental figure you can go to for everything. This person is in your life to help you cope with and recover from brain health challenges.

Vulnerability is a tool that can be used to build deeper bonds. It gives us the opportunity to bear our souls and speak our truths to those who will listen nonjudgmentally. Through this process of trust building, we break down the stigma of brain health one small step at a time. As Dr. Brown puts it, "Trust is a product of vulnerability that grows over time and requires work, attention, and full engagement."

CHAPTER 10

YOU HAVE TO CHANGE YOUR PERSPECTIVE

There are times when life doesn't feel fair. If you're anything like I was, you might feel like your feelings of anxiety and depression are undeserved. I hated my anxiety and depression, and maybe you do, too. You didn't ask for this burden. You have so many other challenges with school, grades, internships, job searches, and your friends, and now you have to worry about improving your brain health.

You might wake up thinking:

"Why does this have to be my reality?"

"What did I do to deserve this?"

"I wish these unbearable feelings would go away!"

"I wish this had never happened."

"I wish I could just feel good again."

I once had those same thoughts. Every morning I started my day with feelings of frustration, desperation, or denial. I hated that I had to deal with emotions other people didn't have to, on top of the normal crap life was throwing at me.

The issue with my thinking, I came to discover, is that it didn't move me forward in any positive way. Days passed by, sure, but I wasn't evolving. Instead, I stayed stuck in my patterns of behavior and thinking. It wasn't until my "aha" moment, when I started to see my situation through a different lens, that my life drastically changed.

I want that lightbulb moment for you, too.

Here's what I figured out: Your brain health challenges, when embraced, can transform you into a better version of yourself. In order for that transformation to occur, you first need to have a new perspective on those challenges. That new outlook is cultivated by *embracing acceptance, finding meaning, and taking ownership.*

Embracing Acceptance

Life is not a gentle and easy journey. The Buddha once said, "Suffering, as a noble truth, is this: Birth is suffering, aging is suffering, sickness is suffering, death is suffering, sorrow and lamentation, pain, grief, and despair are suffering." In other words, suffering is a part of life, and at some point we are going to feel emotions we wish we didn't have to feel. No one is immune to that.

Anxiety and depression most often fall into the category of emotions we wish we could avoid. They can be demoralizing, frustrating, and painful. If this resonates with you and you notice yourself getting frustrated or angry because you still feel these emotions, then it's important to be aware of that in order to move forward.

The first step in changing your perspective is by accepting what is. Acceptance is cultivated through becoming aware of how we feel about people, places, and situations.

Now, before you throw the book across the room, thinking, "Acceptance!? He wants to talk about acceptance. What type of BS is that? I don't want to accept how I feel!" I want you to consider something. Has the way that you've thought about your situation made you any more well off?

If you're like I was, upon reflection, the answer is no. Your feelings of anger, self-hatred, denial, avoidance, frustration, resentment, and self-loathing aren't doing anything for you. They're keeping you stuck in the same old place. You hate the way you feel, but because you wish things were different, you cause yourself more suffering. This occurs because your outward desires are in conflict with your inner reality.

Your thoughts and feelings about your current situation can trap you in a vicious cycle of thinking.

Imagine sitting beside a stream of running water. If you were to place rocks one by one across the stream, creating a dam that didn't allow water through, what would happen? Water would build up and swirl around. A pool would form, and nothing would be able to get through. The water would eventually spill over in all directions, following the path of least resistance. This would disrupt the path the stream was already on. But, if you were to remove the rocks, water would flow again in the direction it was always intended to go, with no resistance.

Your thoughts and feelings are like the stream of water, endless in nature. You sitting beside the stream, watching the water and dam, is like the process of observing your own thoughts and feelings. Simply observing helps build awareness of your thoughts and feelings. The dam is like your resistance to ideas and situations. The overflowing water is like your unchecked behavior. The water finds the path of least resistance, just like it's human nature to desire the path of least resistance or suffering. Acceptance is like the willingness to intentionally remove the dam of resistance by systematically dismantling it, allowing the water to run freely in the direction it was always intended to go.

By becoming aware of the negative beliefs you have about a certain situation, you can begin to cultivate acceptance toward it. You can begin to accept that at times you just won't feel great. It doesn't mean that you'll succumb to whatever you're struggling with, but if you come to terms with it, you can move forward. Constantly wishing things were different isn't going to get you very far.

For me, I stayed stuck because I couldn't accept that I had a new norm with OCD. I was in denial of my new reality and wanted things to go back to the way they were before. It wasn't until I became aware of my resistant thinking and started to accept my new norm that I could move forward. This acceptance will be critically important for you, as it's what will ultimately set you free and opens the door to growth.

So how do I cultivate self-awareness?

For one thing, start a meditation practice. Take time a few days a week, for ten minutes at a time, to simply sit with your thoughts and feelings and notice them. Journaling in the morning or evening is also a great way to start to better understand yourself. You might also consider asking for feedback on how you are progressing with your brain health from people who genuinely care about you and want to see you flourish.

One caveat: In order for these methods to be effective and for growth to occur, you have to be open to the feedback you receive. If you constantly reject new information or perspectives as they're presented to you, growth will be nearly impossible. For that reason, an open mind is a key ingredient to cultivating awareness.

Finding Meaning

You will face challenges in your life that will test you in every way possible. These trials will leave you feeling hopeless, lost, and fearful. You might even begin to ask yourself, "What's the point to life?"

In these tough moments, it's important to search for some meaning that pushes you forward in a positive way. You should start by asking, "What's something I can learn from the anxiety and depression I'm feeling?" You could even consider becoming involved in a nonprofit, support group, or business once you recover. Think about who in your life could benefit from hearing your story after you recover. Will this challenging time in your life make you a better person for your friends and family? The answer to these types of questions will give you extra motivation to move forward, even when you don't feel like dealing with your anxiety and depression.

Having a sense of meaning serves you because it changes your perspective about what you're going through. It's no longer a negative, random, unfortunate fate that you've been sentenced to, but rather a gift. A challenge that in the moment you wish you didn't have to deal with, maybe, but something you'll be able to share with others as you recover.

HAVING A SENSE OF MEANING SERVES YOU BECAUSE IT CHANGES YOUR PERSPECTIVE ABOUT WHAT YOU'RE GOING THROUGH.

Think about all of the wisdom and insight you'll gain after you've grown and evolved from what you're experiencing now.

A great example of creating meaning through your struggles comes from a friend of mine, Julia, who founded a company called BroglieBox. Her company is a brain health subscription box filled with educational resources and evidence-based tools to help maintain your brain health. She was inspired to found the company after experiencing her own brain health challenges as a young adult and losing her brother, Justin, to suicide when he was just twenty-four years old.

Justin's passing inspired her to imagine a new way to support people struggling with stress and wanting to maintain their brain health in today's hectic and often impersonal world. She did not choose for her brother to commit suicide, and she didn't choose to struggle with depression and anxiety, but she did choose how to respond. She still goes to therapy three times a month to maintain her brain health and work through her traumas, all while running a company.

Taking Ownership

When we find ourselves in undesirable situations, we might believe it's not our fault, and therefore not our responsibility to have to deal with it. I certainly believed that, and you might, too. The reality is that we're all responsible for experiences that aren't our fault all the time. According to Mark Manson, author of *The Subtle Art of Not Giving a F*ck*, fault is past tense. Responsibility is present tense. Fault results from choices that have already been made, while responsibility results from the choices you're currently making.

In his words, "Many people may be to blame for your unhappiness, but nobody is ever responsible for your unhappiness but you." This is because you always get to choose how you respond to situations in your life. It might not be your fault that you're feeling depressed, anxious, or stressed out. You might not have chosen for your parents to get divorced. You might not choose to have a sibling commit suicide. You might not choose to have been sexually assaulted. You might not choose to have been discriminated against. You might not choose to be diagnosed with a chronic brain disorder. None of these situations are your fault.

You *do* get to choose how you respond, though.

Do you go to therapy to work through your traumas in a healthy way? Do you take time to practice self-love? Do you make the effort to seek justice? And let me be very clear: I am in no way saying to brush off trauma. What I am saying is that you don't have to let trauma define you for the rest of your life, the same way I actively work every day to not let my brain disorder define me. You get to choose how you respond. That response will dictate the direction you take your life.

I share this with you because I prolonged my suffering for far too long, believing my brain disorder was not my fault and therefore not my responsibility. It wasn't until my perspective changed that I realized no one but me was going to get me well, and that required actually doing the ERP therapy that was assigned to me. Sure, my psychologist could tell me all the right things to do, but if I refused to do them because I didn't feel I had to, then who was to blame for my suffering? Me.

Your brain health challenges can teach you. In recovering from them, you'll learn more about yourself than you could ever imagine. You'll grow and develop as a wiser, more compassionate, and stronger individual. Change your perspective, so you can open the door to your gift. Who knows? The meaning you find might guide you to become the next big brain health advocate helping millions of people across the globe.

CHAPTER 11

CREATE A MEANINGFUL GOAL

In 2016, I started a company with a friend of mine, Christian W., in North Carolina called Great Minds. The company's mission was to help others become the best version of themselves. Our motto was, "You don't have to be great to start. You just need to start, to be great," which was a riff on a quote from one of our role models at the time, Zig Ziglar. To the outside world, I'm sure we looked like a couple kids who were underqualified to be giving life advice. To me, though, it was everything.

Seriously, though. It was literally my lifeline.

At the same time I was starting a business with a good friend of mine, I was also dealing with the rollercoaster of depression, anxiety, and suicidal thoughts. My OCD had kicked in hard. Most days I woke up exhausted or didn't want to get out of bed. Life felt pointless. But the one thing that would always get me out of bed was the business. I loved the goal we had to help other people and the idea that we could build something from scratch. When we were working on the company, my symptoms would temporarily subside. When we weren't, the symptoms would flood back into my consciousness. In a way, the business was an escape from reality. It was an escape from my brain. But it also gave every day meaning at a time when I felt like I was holding on by a thread. I was no longer just floating through life. Every day, we had tasks to complete and a meaningful goal we were chasing: to change lives!

The same applies to you. Meaningful goals matter for everyone. And please don't confuse "finding your purpose" with chasing a meaningful goal. To me, "finding your purpose" sounds a little daunting, and how can you really measure when you've found it? Instead, identify what really lights you up. What's the one thing you always find time for? It's something you want to get better at. It's something you want to chase and explore. Chances are, it's something you're passionate about. And where passion and a desire for growth intersect is where you'll find a meaningful goal.

MEANINGFUL GOALS MATTER FOR EVERYONE.

Maybe you really enjoy painting, and your goal is to get your artwork displayed in a local art gallery. Maybe you love physical training, so you train for five months leading up to a Spartan Race. Maybe you have a passion for photography and you're trying to start a small wedding photography business. It could be managing an Instagram page that posts about civil rights. It could be working to organize and grow a book club because you love classic literature. It could be working on that EP you've always wanted to put out because you're a hip-hop artist.

This meaningful goal is an expression of you in one form or another. So embrace it and let it fill space in your daily life. That will enrich your good days and make it easier, if only slightly, to get through the dark days, too.

Below I've laid out some simple steps to help you create a meaningful goal. Remember, you can make it as big or as small as you want it to be. It's yours to pursue.

Setting Meaningful Goals

Setting a meaningful goal for yourself can be a little daunting. That's why it's important to reflect. To start, ask yourself a few questions:

- What gave you the most energy in your life this past year?
- What was a pain point from the past year?

- What moments made you proud of yourself this year?
- Who did you admire this year?
- What did you want to learn more about in your free time this year?
- What activities did you loath doing?

The goal here is to start to identify potential areas of interest, while weeding out areas that don't light you up.

Free Write

Free writing is really helpful and something I do whenever I feel stuck trying to come up with an idea. This is a nonjudgmental approach where you allow yourself to brain-dump everything in your head, starting with a few simple questions. Those questions could include:

- What do I want to learn more about this year?
- What would my ideal future look like a year from now?
- What topics interest me the most?
- What are my strengths?

As an example, back in 2016 I really wanted to learn more about entrepreneurship. Business was a topic that always interested me, and now that I felt like an adult, I wanted to start to learn more about that topic. What had given me the most energy in the previous year was reading about entrepreneurs and people who had gone out and started their own businesses. It was exciting to me and gave me energy, no matter how I was feeling. Nowadays what interests me the most is what impacts globalization, AI, work environments, racial equality, and the increased pressures to perform at work and school are having on college students and society as a whole. Your interests could be sports related, music related, technology related, and so on.

Asking What For?

Your answer is going to feel big and vague at first, and that's okay. Starting out broad allows you to brain-dump all of the exciting things you *could* pursue this year, without the pressure of needing to have a plan. A broad example could be, "I want to be more confident." That's great! This big, vague goal can be more refined.

Let's say you've decided your broad goal is to be more confident this year. Let's take it a step further. Ask yourself, "What for? Why do I want to be more confident?" Maybe it's because you're working up the courage to speak to someone you've always liked. It could be because you want to become a better public speaker. It could be because you want to start showing off your artwork to other students on campus. Or you want to take on a leadership role in your fraternity or sorority but haven't been confident about your abilities in the past. Try and define why you want what you want.

Refine Your Goal Using SMART

Now that you've brain-dumped and created a broad goal for yourself, it's time to take it a step further using the acronym SMART.

Specific:

Your goal should state exactly what you want to do this year, with as much detail as possible. You want to give yourself the gift of a specific goal, so that once you've achieved it, you know.

Using the example above, you could want to feel more confident, so you take on a leadership role on campus or at work. A more specific example would then be, "Read one book on cultivating self-confidence and one book on leadership in the next two months. I will then take on a leadership role for Student Government."

Measurable:

Your goal needs to be quantified, either numerically or descriptively. You need some measurement that describes exactly when you have achieved it. If your goal is to take on a leadership role, attach some sort of numerical value to it to help quantify your efforts, like "Read two books on confidence and leadership. Attend the next five Student Government meetings."

Action-Oriented:

There should always be an action tied to your specific goal. This will force you to get started, even if you are nervous or scared. If your goal is to be more of a leader in your fraternity, you're not identifying an action you can take. Instead, saying something like, "Help one member in my fraternity a week on their mental health" is an action you can take that makes you a leader in that regard.

If your meaningful goal scares you a little bit, that's a good thing. It means you're being taken out of your comfort zone and forcing yourself to grow. Don't let fear deter you. Just get started. Learn to become comfortable with being uncomfortable. That's where the growth happens.

Realistic:

Your goal needs to be based somewhat on previous performance. If you've always been a shy person and never taken on a leadership role, it might be unrealistic to think you'll get voted to be Student Government president on your first attempt, especially if you're new to the organization. Knowing your past performances allows you to understand your abilities, while pushing you outside of your comfort zone.

A more realistic goal might be to finish the two books you've identified and then take on a smaller leadership role inside an organization. Even if going for president is what you desire long-term, a stepping-stone leadership role is exactly what you need to learn more about leading people. You also have a much higher chance of getting it, which will give you momentum and confidence to try for a bigger leadership role the next time around.

Your goal should stretch you outside of your comfort zone, while simultaneously being realistic. If you're setting a meaningful goal that really stretches you, there is a chance that you won't completely accomplish that goal. You might accomplish some variation of that goal, which is something to be proud of. Don't get down on yourself. You know you're on the right path when your goal is hard to accomplish. Modify and revise as you go. Remember, your goal is supposed to motivate and excite you, not make you feel down.

Time Bound:

Your goal should have a timeline attached to it. This gives you a deadline. It also forces you to take a little bit of action toward that goal every day. If your goal is to take on a leadership role in Student Government and you know those roles will be voted on in four months, this gives you a clear date to work toward.

Using that example, the first thing you'd need to do is join Student Government and start attending the meetings. Then you'd have the next four months to read the books you've identified and start to get your name out there as a candidate. The clearer you are on the date, the better. It will motivate you every day to take an action toward your goal.

CHAPTER 12

LET GO OF THE PAST

In my work as a speaker and a coach, I get the chance to meet a lot of people who struggle with anxiety and depression. I've noticed that so many people beat themselves up over past mistakes and perceived failures. They point back to moments in their life and wish things were different. Or they look at their lives and become sad or frustrated because things haven't gone the way they hoped. This might be the same for you.

Maybe you just moved back in with your parents because you didn't have the grades you needed to stay in school. You might be upset because you're a senior and feel like you didn't make enough friends while in college, and now you think it's too late. Perhaps you wish you would've been involved in more clubs or activities. Maybe you feel embarrassed by something you did while at school that you wish you could take back. Whatever it is you're holding onto, I know these feelings of regret, frustration, and sadness can be haunting.

People who struggle with anxiety and depression tend to be incredibly hard on themselves. For some reason, the voice in our heads seems to be a little louder and more critical. Somewhere deep inside our brains, we don't believe the anxiety and depression we struggle with on a daily basis is a valid enough reason to have setbacks. We believe that we should be stronger, and when we don't meet that expectation, the self-critic chimes in to give its two cents.

In this chapter, you're going to learn to give yourself permission to let go of the past, in three easy steps. You will change your relationship with failure, forgive yourself, and then take action.

Get into a Growth Mindset

Humans make mistakes every single day. Yet all of us fear making mistakes because deep down inside we fear judgment and rejection. In your life, it is 100 percent guaranteed that you will make a mistake, too. The key to overcoming failure is recognizing that everybody makes mistakes. You are not alone, and I promise you somebody has made the same mistake as you.

It's time to shift your perspective to a growth mindset. A growth mindset is the belief that you can improve your intelligence, ability, and performance over time by learning from your mistakes. When you come to understand that lasting growth stems from setbacks and failures, you turn perceived negative situations into positive ones. This puts you in control!

Armed with this new perspective, you never need to get down on yourself in moments where you feel like you've failed. Instead of chalking it up to a failure, a person with a growth mindset asks themselves, "What did I learn from this situation, so I can grow from it in the future? What can I do differently this next time around to get a more desirable outcome?" That shift in mindset is enough to put the control and power back with you, because you now get to choose how you see the situation and how you react.

Forgiveness Sets You Free

You might be thinking, "I get what this guy is saying about the growth mindset thing, but my whole life is a mess. I can't seem to get anything right. My anxiety and depression sucks, and I can't get past it. I've messed everything up. It's too late for me. I've ruined my future."

I get why you might believe that, but this is one of the many lies we all tell ourselves. When we are in that dark place, we believe we'll stay there forever. We believe whatever it is we messed up is the worst thing ever. You might believe you're a failure and that your future is irreparable. I'm here to tell you that's not true. Bryan Stevenson once said, "I believe that each person is more than the worst thing they've done." You are so much more than any of your recent or past mistakes. No matter what you've done or said, it's okay. You have a bright future ahead of you, but first you need to forgive yourself.

First, notice any resentment you hold toward your anxiety, depression, and yourself. Acknowledge what you are feeling. Acknowledge that you wish things were different. Allow whatever feelings that bubble up to be present. Don't run from them or deny them. You might even give them a nod and say, "I see you there. Thanks for being present with me."

Then ask yourself if you'd be willing to forgive yourself if it meant you would have a better, brighter future? Sit with that question. Allow thoughts to bubble up again without wrestling with them, trying to change them, or suppressing them. You might notice the self-critic yelling at you, calling you a failure. Let that voice be, without turning away from it.

Next, I want you to do something you might've never done before. I want you to look yourself in the mirror, lock eyes with yourself, and tell yourself: "I forgive you."

I WANT YOU TO LOOK YOURSELF IN THE MIRROR, LOCK EYES WITH YOURSELF, AND TELL YOURSELF: "I FORGIVE YOU."

Then let it all out. Forgive yourself for everything. Forgive yourself for not performing in school. Forgive yourself for struggling with depression and anxiety. Forgive yourself for not being where you want to be in life. Forgive yourself for the friends you wish you'd made. Forgive yourself for not feeling confident in who you are. Forgive your parents for their divorce. Forgive the person who bullied you in the past. Forgive the friend who turned their back on you and caused you pain. Forgive yourself for that embarrassing thing you did. Forgive yourself for the worst thing you ever did. Forgive yourself for the missed opportunities. Forgive it all. This might feel foreign at first. It might be hard to forgive yourself right away, but give it time. Just like anything in life, forgiveness is a skill that is built over time through intention and repetition.

By consciously bringing forgiveness to the forefront, you put space between whatever struggle you're going through and yourself. You bring that guilt out of the dark, into the light where you can see it clearly. You look it in the face and say, "Enough. I forgive you. Now it's time to do something about this pain."

Once you've truly forgiven yourself, it's possible to heal and move forward, and in doing so, you no longer have to operate under the weight you carry from relentlessly criticizing yourself every day. Of course, this is a process, and takes time and effort. It won't happen overnight, but by beginning to accept that you're human and thus imperfect, you won't be defined by your depression and anxiety anymore. You are ready for a new beginning.

Action Is the Antidote

Once you've forgiven yourself, it's time to take action. If your depression or anxiety is interfering with you leading the life you desire, then start there. Schedule an appointment with a brain health professional who can help you begin to feel better.

With the support of a trained professional, you can begin to slowly and gently build the life you want. You'll set small, bite-size SMART goals. You might wish you exercised more, so start by doing three walks (measurable) around campus a week (time bound). Maybe you want to go back to school (realistic), so start by taking two online courses to get your general credits (action-oriented). Maybe you wish you had more friends, so start by going to one social gathering and meeting one new person (measurable). These steps might feel difficult at first, but with commitment and repetition they'll become your new norm.

The reality is that letting go is a verb. Forgiving yourself is a verb. No amount of positive thinking or positive affirmations will build you back up. You need to move away from your past in order to build a new future. If you want the life you've always yearned for, you have to let go of any past shortcomings. Forgive yourself, because you deserve that.

You are the architect of your life. It's time to build.

CHAPTER 13

MEANINGFUL WORK IS NOT EVERYTHING

When I first entered into the workforce, I was obsessed with the idea that I was going to "grind" nonstop to build the life of my dreams. I wanted to make tons of money and have a job that was aligned with my life purpose. Then I started to actually work, and I quickly realized that my job wasn't filling me up the way I expected it to. It wasn't aligned with my purpose of changing the world and doing great things. As a result, I spent a lot of time struggling. If I wasn't doing what I was meant to do, then what was the point in life?

This thought process was both narrowly focused and dangerous. It created pressure to find work that was meaningful, which in turn put a lot of unnecessary stress on me. It also created a sense of lack in my life, where I felt like I was missing something. This destroyed the opportunity to feel grateful for even having a job. Despite having a great job with benefits, time off, and opportunities for growth, I felt like a failure. And feeling like a failure, over time, was wearing on my mind and hurting how I perceived myself. It nearly killed every bit of confidence I had and created a lot of anxiety because I felt like life was passing me by and I hadn't changed the world. It wasn't until a few years had passed that I saw the errors in my thinking.

For decades, the American dream was informally defined as having a stable job, being a homeowner, and raising a family. Then, somewhere along the way, our culture shifted and decided that work couldn't just pay the bills, it also had to have some type of deeper meaning. However, finding meaningful work can be extremely difficult, everyone has a different idea of what qualifies as "meaningful work," and placing too much emphasis on what you do for a living can have impacts on your relationships with your family and friends, and your physical and mental health.

Oftentimes what gets forgotten in the conversation about finding meaningful work is that pursuing meaningful work requires privilege. If in your current job you earn minimum wage and there's little or no room for growth with your employer, then it's unlikely that you perceive your current career path as meaningful. For that reason, it's insensitive and short-sighted to expect that every single person should be seeking meaning in their work. For most people, work is a means to put clothes on their backs, food on the table, and a roof over their head. To demand that your work have meaning implies that other basic burdens of life don't apply to you. This is a privilege that not everyone gets to enjoy.

I'm not suggesting that searching for meaningful work or trying to change the world are bad moves. Rather, I'm suggesting that you consider a different, broader perspective that allows you to see value in your work and be grateful no matter what your job is. From my experience, this will drastically improve your brain health and save you from spending your life discontented because your work isn't oozing with deep meaning.

The Culprit

In Western cultures and especially in the US, we've created a culture around needing to find meaningful work. The reality is that a large portion of us might not have even considered "finding meaningful work" important if someone else hadn't told us that was the thing to do. Our culture is fixated on doing more, being more productive, and working longer hours. We've been led to believe that the harder we work, the more money we'll make, which will result in bigger houses, nicer cars, and better clothes, which will make us happier. What we fail to see is that our material desires don't fill us up long-term. Working longer hours for the bigger house, nicer car, and better clothes doesn't always translate to contentment and fulfillment. As we talked about earlier, work burnout is a real thing. No matter the situation, no job or level of pay is worth the deterioration of your brain health. Always put your health first and your job second.

The Dalai Lama once said, "When it comes to dealing with greed, one thing that is quite characteristic is that although it arrives by the desire to obtain something, it is not satisfied by obtaining. Therefore, it becomes sort of limitless, sort of bottomless, and that leads to trouble. One interesting thing about greed is that although the underlying motive is to seek satisfaction, the irony is that even after obtaining the object of your desire, you are still not satisfied."

This is why it's important to think about what you value. What you value is what you inevitably prioritize. For example, if you value working over spending time with your friends, you will inevitably spend more time at your job and less time with your friends. This could have ramifications in the form of damaged or lost friendships. You can spend your whole life working, and if you have no one to enjoy it with, then what was the point of it all? Furthermore, your priorities change over time. If you feel fulfilled by your family or social life, then being connected to your work may not—and doesn't need to be—of utmost importance. For that reason, it's unrealistic to expect that your job will check all the boxes of meaning all of the time. If you only value your work, what happens if that work abruptly gets taken away from you?

Your Job Isn't the Only Way to Find Meaning

There are so many other ways to contribute to the world other than your work. The reality is that, for some people, a job is a job. And working your job is a way to make money so that you can contribute in other ways like giving back via charity or volunteering. In fact, an early 2000s study discovered that two parts of the brain, the VTA and the subgenual area, both considered "reward" centers, were activated when participants placed the interests of others before themselves. Research also found that volunteering improved the health of volunteers both physically and emotionally. Therefore, you might find more meaning in volunteer work for an organization that champions a cause you support, or maybe you donate regularly toward a charitable cause.

It's important to consider what function your work is serving in your life, and it's okay if your work isn't the sole source of meaning in your world. Chalking up your job as a job doesn't make you a loser or a failure. Not everybody needs to be the next Steve Jobs or Elon Musk. If your job is just a job, that's okay. If the income you make from that job allows you to enjoy your life by spending time with friends and family, and doesn't cause you too much stress, what's wrong with that?!

Helping Others Helps You

Ultimately, what I discovered early in my career is that striving to make more money didn't create higher levels of happiness. Striving to get promotions and more prestigious titles at my corporate job didn't make me happier. Oftentimes, my promotions did more harm than good for my brain health by causing increased levels of stress and anxiety. Sure, the money helped me live slightly more comfortable, but I didn't achieve a new level of happiness. In the end, damage to my peace of mind was not worth the paycheck.

Where I have found deep meaning and contentment consistently, though, is through my advocacy work with brain health. I have traveled all over the country, stayed in cheap hotels, eaten pizza by the slice, tossed and turned before speeches, flown on Spirit Airlines from coast to coast, sandwiched in a middle seat, and spent countless hours listening to people across the globe share their brain health struggles with me. Every second of struggle has been worth it because helping people feels good. What I've discovered is that deep inside each and every one of us is a compassion and love we didn't even know we had. When you help somebody, you help yourself because it feels good to help another human. We lose sight of this, though, in our pursuit for money and status.

WHEN YOU HELP SOMEBODY, YOU HELP YOURSELF.

As you prepare to graduate from college, I would encourage you to consider these questions: Do you think the career path you're taking will be good for your brain health? Are you doing it for the money because you think the money will bring you happiness? Where in your life can you help others?

PART 4

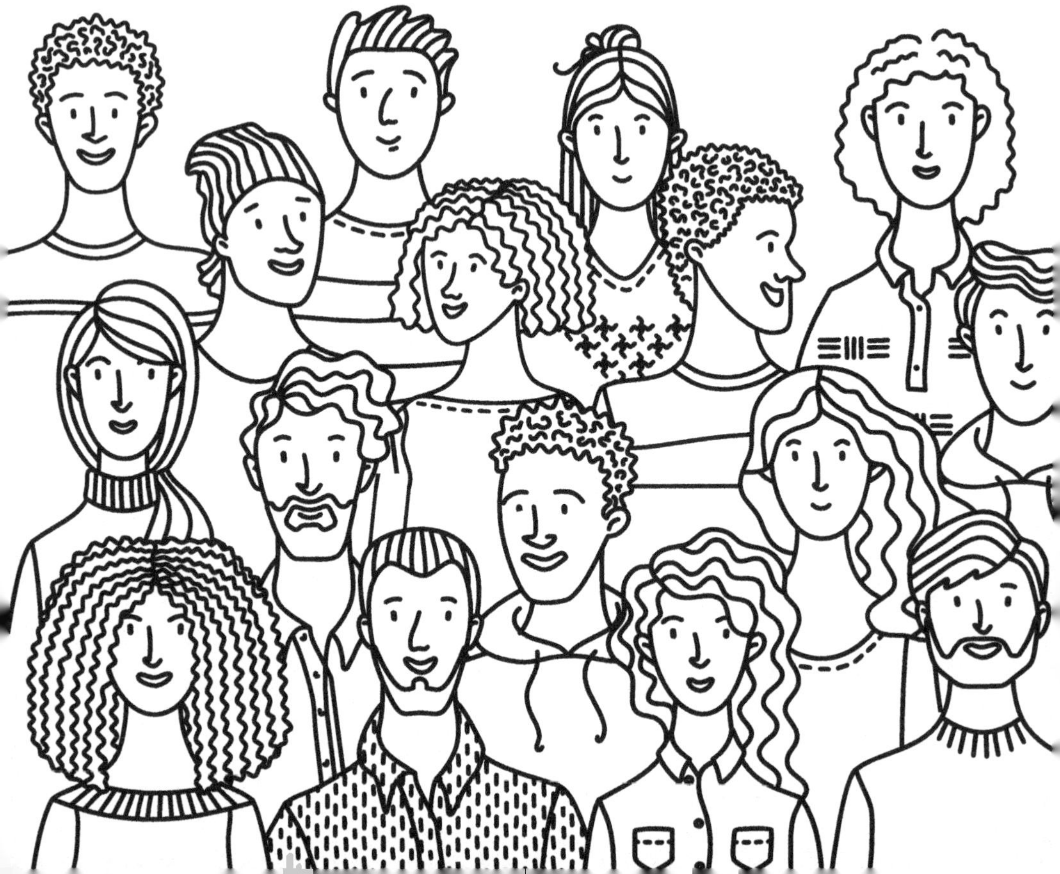

CHAPTER 14

CREATE A ROUTINE

Think of your routine as the foundation of your brain health blueprint. As you're planning out your routine, we'll focus on five areas to promote positive brain health, to help you thrive academically and socially: sleep, meditation, exercise, rest, and reading.

Sleep Is Priority Number One

Sleep is the most important thing you can give your brain and body. Therefore, as you start planning out your routine, consider sleep the anchor of your schedule. That means deciding on what time you want to start winding down for the night, what time you want to close your eyes, what time you want to start waking up, and what time you actually get out of bed to start your day.

As a general rule of thumb, you should schedule an hour before bed to start your wind-down process. Focus on doing simple activities that don't require any critical thinking. I recommend reading a book. Try a novel or something that's not too information-heavy.

Next, pick the time you actually want to go to bed. For me, I want to close my eyes by 11:00 p.m.

After that, you need to decide on your wake-up time. Plenty of people, especially in American culture, will tell you that the most successful individuals get up bright and early. That works for some people, but not everyone. When I tried waking up super early for a while in college, it ended up making me feel tired and groggy the entire day.

Choose a time that maximizes your sleep. For example, if you have 7:00 a.m. classes (which is ridiculously early in my opinion), you should be winding down by 9:00 p.m. and in bed by 10:00 p.m., so you can wake up at 6:00 a.m. Give yourself an hour in the morning to slowly wake up, drink water, eat a little food, and then head to class.

Meditation

From personal experience, I would recommend scheduling ten minutes of meditation in the morning as a part of your morning routine. Studies have shown that you only need ten minutes of meditation to reap the benefits, and this can be a tone setter for the rest of your day. On days when I meditate in the morning, I am calmer, more focused, more relaxed, and more compassionate. I notice that my anxiety levels are lower and my brain feels better. Give your brain the mental exercise it deserves by making meditation a staple in your daily routine, and do it first thing in the morning so you don't get distracted and skip it. More on this to come.

Exercise

Plan time to move your body every day. I work out in the mornings because my body feels most awake then, and it fits best with my work schedule. Your exercise schedule might look different. Aim to exercise three to four times a week at a time when your body feels most awake, to release endorphins and decrease tension. In addition, schedule time to take a walk outside at least once a day, maybe after classes, to help naturally release stress and tension in the body.

Siestas Aren't Just for Spaniards

When I studied in Spain while in college, I had the opportunity to participate in the Spanish culture of siestas. If you're unfamiliar with the term, a *siesta* is a period in the day when Spaniards take a break from work, go home to eat a big meal with their families, and then rest before going back to work. It was an experience I loved and something that has done wonders for my brain health.

Our American capitalist culture has put such an emphasis on productivity that we look at taking breaks and resting as a negative thing. This is total BS and a belief you should scrap right now. The reality is that you are not a robot. You are a human. Humans get tired, experience fatigue, and need rest. Resting and taking a nap for twenty to thirty minutes in the middle of the day is great for your brain. It helps provide natural energy and can relieve feelings of stress and anxiety. Schedule time to rest each day, in the afternoon and evening. As an example, take thirty minutes, from 2:30 to 3:00 p.m., to rest your eyes. Later on, after a full day of studying, rest in the evening before getting dinner. Scheduling rest is so important for your brain health.

THE REALITY IS THAT YOU ARE NOT A ROBOT. YOU ARE A HUMAN.

Read

Lastly, take time each day to read and think. In our American culture, we are accustomed to the idea that we should fill every waking hour with work and *doing*. You wake up, immediately dart to class, stay on campus for the whole day, only stopping for lunch, then dart back to your room, do homework, study, play video games, eat dinner, and then sleep. Repeat, repeat, repeat.

The issue with always doing is that we never take the time to stop, read something we enjoy, and then think about it. Yet studies show that reading things we enjoy has psychological benefits for our brain. As you build out your routine, I would encourage you to schedule time each day to read something that's stimulating to you. Then take a little bit of time to think about what you've read. In those moments of quiet, you might experience clarity you didn't expect to find. Worst case, it's an opportunity for your brain to unwind, bringing more calm into your life.

Creating a routine around the five core areas mentioned above will help promote positive brain health. Scheduling ample amounts of sleep should be at the core of your routine, and everything else in your day should fit around that.

CHAPTER 15

GIVE YOURSELF THE GIFT OF SLEEP

In college, I never gave myself the quality of sleep my brain needed to function at its highest level. I was never on a consistent sleeping schedule. One day I was pulling an all-nighter for an exam, and the next night I was drinking to celebrate the fact that the exam was over. I still remember the day I convinced myself sleep wasn't important. It was after two weeks of getting only about four hours of sleep per night. During that time, I managed to complete homework assignments, take quizzes, and party with friends—all while getting almost no sleep. Sleep was overrated, I thought.

It wasn't until many years later that my poor sleep habits caught up with me. As I tried to perform at my job and cope with anxiety and depression, I noticed I was exhausted. My brain hurt. I couldn't focus and I didn't have energy. Eventually, I realized there was a correlation between my feelings of happiness, focus, and calm and the amount of quality sleep I gifted myself. I started to prioritize sleep, which directly impacted how my brain felt.

From the students I've polled in my travels, I've observed that most seem to get an average of four to six hours of sleep a night. You might fall into that category because you don't believe that sleep is important. Or maybe you believe sleep is important, but you don't prioritize it in your day. From your perspective, there are other priorities, like staying up late studying for homework and exams, hanging out with friends, playing video games until two in the morning, or partying. In addition, you feel pressure to perform academically to make your parents happy and set yourself up for the future. You might be juggling a full course load, a part-time job, leadership roles, extracurriculars, and a social life.

Whatever the reason, skimping on sleep can cause you to wake up with zero energy. No sleep combined with a packed schedule can interfere with how you feel big-time. You might notice your mood is off, you're more irritable, and you feel totally unmotivated. I'm here to tell you that no amount of coffee will help.

If you're going to be successful, both academically and with your brain health, then you have to make sleep the most important thing you do all day. Sleep is foundational to your brain health and will dictate your success in life. Don't believe people who say they blow off sleep and get by just fine. They don't.

As a culture, we love to be busy and productive, often at the expense of our health. This has become so normalized that people wear their worn-out, stressed out, sleep-deprived status like it's a badge of honor. Don't buy into that nonsense. If you're going to take care of your brain and properly manage symptoms of depression and anxiety, good sleep habits have to come first.

GOOD SLEEP HABITS HAVE TO COME FIRST.

The reality is that twenty-four hours is ample time to accomplish anything you want to in a day. You can have friends, excel in school, and work a job while also gifting yourself quality sleep.

The Benefits

According to the National Sleep Foundation's 2018 Sleep in America poll, one in three adults in the United States has increased anxiety due to not getting enough sleep. Fortunately, you have the ability to recover from poor sleep. It starts by improving your sleep hygiene and mentality about sleep. Below are some of the benefits that you get from accumulating quality sleep over time.

Lower stress: When our bodies are sleep deficient, they go into a state of stress. The body is put on high alert, which causes high blood pressure and the production of stress hormones. Stress hormones make it difficult to fall asleep. Conversely, when you allow yourself more sleep, this reduces the production of stress hormones and gives your body and mind the opportunity to relax and fall into a deeper sleep.

Less inflammation: Lack of sleep raises stress hormone levels in the body, which in turn increases the level of inflammation in the body. This increased inflammation puts you at greater risk for heart-related conditions, as well as depression. There are studies emerging in the medical field that indicate inflammation can be linked to the likelihood of you becoming depressed.

Improved memory: Researchers have found that quality sleep plays an important role in a process called memory consolidation. While your body is resting during sleep, your brain is busy processing the day and making connections between events, feelings, and memories. Getting deep sleep is critical, as it helps you remember and process things better.

Reduced risk of depression: Sleep has an impact on chemical regulation in your body, including serotonin. Ensuring you get between seven and ten hours of sleep each night may lower your risk of depression.

Healthy Sleep Tips

Creating healthy sleep habits can make a huge difference in your overall health and quality of life. *Sleep hygiene*, as it's referred to, is the process of creating and implementing healthy sleep habits. By creating and then refining your sleep hygiene, you can drastically improve your health. It is important to know that each person is different. For example, I feel most refreshed when I get nine to ten hours of sleep, while others may only need seven to feel alert and at their best.

Create and stick to a sleep schedule: Sleep should be your number one priority. Everything else you do during your waking hours should be scheduled around it. Create a sleep schedule that includes a bedtime and a wake-up time. By being consistent this way, you'll help regulate your body's internal clock, and that could help you stay asleep longer at night. Your schedule should include weekends as well, which can be difficult in college or as a young adult due to your social life. Try to stick to your schedule six nights out of seven, which might mean making Friday or Saturday your going-out night.

Practice a relaxing bedtime ritual: Finding a relaxing activity to do an hour or so before bed is critical to developing sound sleep hygiene. The activity should be conducted away from bright light or the blue light created by screens. Avoid activities that will cause you to feel excitement, stress, or anxiety (like responding to work or school emails). Diving into a good book is a solid idea. If your living situation involves a roommate, see if you can get them onboard to be more low-key Sunday through Wednesday or Thursday night.

Befriend napping: Throw out any old beliefs you have about taking naps. Grabbing a quick twenty-minute power nap between classes or during a break has been shown to be more effective and refreshing than drinking a cup of coffee in the afternoon. People who take time for a quick nap show much lower levels of stress, improved memory and mood, and better cognitive function.

I personally have found twenty- to thirty-minute naps help increase my energy and focus. In addition, naps simply make my brain feel better. They help reduce my headaches, fatigue, and anxiety. Don't buy into the idea that naps are for lazy people or that you don't have enough time to nap.

Exercise daily: Exercise has a host of benefits for your overall health, including improved sleep. Vigorous exercise that gets your heart rate up is best, but a walk around the neighborhood can help as well. The goal is to use mindfulness to be present and focus on the activity you are doing.

This will reduce the likelihood of racing thoughts before bed and release endorphins to help you relax.

Evaluate your room: Your room's main function should be to support good sleep, so plan your room out accordingly. Don't keep a TV in your room, as this will encourage falling asleep with the TV on, which impacts the quality of your sleep. Do keep your bedroom cool. The ideal bedroom temperature for sleep is 67 degrees Fahrenheit. Aim to have your room between 67 and 72 degrees. You want your room to be as quiet as possible. If you're like me and live on a busy street, try using a fan coupled with earplugs to drown out external sounds. Finally, your bedroom should be as dark as possible. Cover up any blinking or power lights and consider using blackout curtains or an eye mask. I sleep with an eye mask that blocks 90 percent of all light. It has immensely improved my quality of sleep.

Sleep on a comfortable mattress and pillows: The average person spends one-third of their life in bed sleeping. For that reason, it's important to invest in a quality mattress and pillows. A quality mattress lasts nine or ten years max. If you're approaching that nine-year mark, it's time to look into buying a new mattress. Additionally, having comfortable pillows will drastically decrease the likelihood of waking up stiff and sore. If you're on a tight budget, like a lot of college students are, invest in a mattress topper to make your bed more comfortable to lie on.

Manage your circadian rhythms: Try to avoid bright light in the evening when you're winding down and expose yourself to sunlight in the morning. Every morning when I wake up, the first thing I do is open up the blinds in our living room to let sunlight in. This helps keep your circadian rhythms in check.

Avoid alcohol, nicotine, and caffeine: Alcohol, nicotine, and caffeine can all disrupt sleep. Alcohol is a sedative and might make you feel sleepy, but once the effect has worn off, you'll wake up in the middle of the night. Caffeine can make you restless and cause racing thoughts as you try to fall asleep. Vaping has made it very convenient to get your nicotine fix while hanging out inside, but all forms of nicotine can mess with quality sleep. As a rule of thumb, try to avoid caffeine after noon and avoid drinking alcohol on nights that you don't plan on going out. Additionally, set parameters around when you allow yourself to vape at night.

Go to another room to wind down: If you're having issues falling asleep at night, get up and go to another room where you can do something relaxing. If you live in a dorm, go out to the lounge or find a quiet corner. The brain associates each room with its different function, one for relaxing and the other for sleeping.

Make your bed a stress-free zone: Lastly, make sure you keep work materials, computers, and televisions out of your sleeping environment. If you live in a dorm or small space and can't keep everything out of your room altogether, at least keep your laptop off your bed and your phone out of reach.

Speak with a sleep specialist: The main theme of this book is to always ask for help! If you're having issues falling asleep at night and it's becoming an ongoing thing, don't hesitate to speak with a doctor or sleep professional. They'll be able to help you put a sleep hygiene plan together.

CHAPTER 16

MOVE YOUR BODY

Most of us have been taught that physical exercise is good for our bodies. Historically, exercise has been used to make our muscles stronger and our physiques more appealing. For those of us living with stress, anxiety, and depression, exercise can improve how your brain feels. In fact, it has been proven that regular exercise profoundly impacts depression, anxiety, ADHD, and other symptoms in a positive way. Exercise can also relieve stress, promote better sleep, and boost overall mood.

If you live more of a sedentary lifestyle, don't enjoy exercise, or don't consider yourself athletic enough to exercise, I understand where you're coming from. The only reason I work out now is for my brain health, because exercise impacts how I feel. Yes, I receive other physical benefits, but frankly, I could care less about that. Endorphins are like ice for my brain: they reduce my headaches, ease tension, and help me feel calm.

THE ONLY REASON I WORK OUT NOW IS FOR MY BRAIN HEALTH, BECAUSE EXERCISE IMPACTS HOW I FEEL.

The good news is that you don't need to be one of those fitness gurus you've probably seen on Instagram, all shredded and whatnot, to get the brain benefits of exercise. Taking a simple walk through your neighborhood or around campus makes a big difference, too. The most important thing is to start doing something. Once you feel the brain benefits, it will naturally become a more important part of your life. Your body will thank you, but your brain will praise you.

To be clear, I am not suggesting that exercise is going to cure a brain disorder or make your depression or anxiety disappear. When I first started experiencing symptoms of depression and anxiety, I tried exercising profusely in an effort to "sweat out" the emotions I was feeling. It didn't work. These days, I notice a stark difference in my feelings of anxiety, stress, and depression on days that I exercise, compared to days that I don't.

Depression and Exercise

According to Harvard Health, exercise can help combat depression. Dr. Michael Craig Miller, assistant professor of psychiatry at Harvard Medical School, states, "It can work as well as antidepressants, although exercise alone isn't enough for someone with severe depression." Additionally, maintaining an exercise schedule can support long-term recovery. That's not to say that feelings of depression won't occur again, but it does mean that you'll already have a tool to use when those feelings arise. From my personal experience, running, lifting weights, playing basketball, and hiking, in conjunction with professional assistance, have been helpful to treat my feelings of depression.

There are a few key reasons exercise is such a good tool to manage depression. When you exercise, there are changes that take place in the brain. You develop new neural pathways that promote feelings of calm and reduce inflammation. Exercise also releases endorphins, which provide a brief euphoric feeling and can be used to briefly suspend pain in the body. If you've ever heard the term "runner's high," this is possible because of endorphins being released by your brain. This feel-good chemical can help lift your mood.

Anxiety, Stress, and Exercise

Exercise is a natural way to reduce your feelings of anxiety. It has the ability to relieve tension and stress. As my fiancée and I always say, "Motion is emotion." If you're feeling anxious, the best thing you can do is get your body moving, whether that's through an intense workout or a walk around the block. While you're moving, try to focus on the movement and feeling of your body instead of zoning out. This will help you stay present, which is the cornerstone of mindfulness.

As an example, you could focus on your breathing while taking a ten-minute walk around your campus. Observe your breath as air moves in and out of your lungs. You can also focus on your feet hitting the ground one at a time. Feel your heel hitting the ground. Notice the sun on your skin. This practice of movement with mindfulness can be very effective in centering your mind and relieving anxiety.

Every single day, I go on brisk walks around my neighborhood to help alleviate anxiety and stress. I walk for as long and as far as I think I need. The entire time, I try to focus on being present. If my mind drifts to thinking about other topics, I try to gently guide it back to what I'm doing in the present moment. By the time I've finished a walk, the tension has left my body and I feel more relaxed.

Other Brain and Mood Benefits of Exercise

More resilience: When you're faced with tough life challenges, exercise can help you cope in a healthy way, rather than resorting to alcohol, drugs, or other negative behaviors that could make your symptoms worse.

Greater confidence: Taking the time to work on your physical appearance can drastically improve your perception of yourself. Completing and accomplishing goals can also be a great way to improve your brain health and your sense of self-worth. As you reach more and more milestones, your confidence will grow because you believe in yourself and your ability to accomplish the goals you set for yourself.

Stronger sense of community: My suggestion would be to always work out with a partner or a group. The sense of community and belonging builds stronger bonds with the people around you. The release of oxytocin creates that sense of unity with those around us, which creates that feeling of "family." It helps facilitate compassion and empathy toward others. Since human beings are social creatures by nature, this gives the brain an extra boost of security. Plus you'll make friends who enjoy healthy habits.

Better performance at school and work: Endorphins not only make you feel good but can be highly beneficial for your cognition. These feel-good chemicals can help keep your brain sharp and fuel creativity and inspiration. You can thank the release of endorphins and neurochemicals like dopamine for keeping us motivated, intrigued, and focused. This, in turn, helps us produce outstanding artwork, music, writing, and inventions, and helps us innovate at school and work. With boosted focus and creativity, you'll find yourself performing better.

Quality sleep: Exercise in the morning or afternoon can help improve your sleep patterns. Endorphins and serotonin affect your overall mood and level of sleepiness. The release of these chemicals helps regulate your circadian rhythm. This naturally occurring bodily function helps you know when it's time to be awake and when it's time to be asleep. When you exercise, these rhythms fall into a more predictable pattern that makes you feel refreshed in the morning and drowsy before bed. If you're someone who prefers to exercise at night, it is recommended that you do more relaxing activities, like yoga or gentle stretching, which also help promote sleep.

Make It a Part of Your Routine

Create a schedule where you work out at the same time every day. The more consistent the schedule, the more likely the workout will happen. Take advantage of the gym on your campus. It's free, and probably not too far from where you spend a good chunk of your day. Pack a gym bag and pop by before or after class or work. If you're the type of person who's 100 percent not working out the second you step into your home, then make sure you avoid that. If sticking with a consistent routine is really a struggle, find a fitness partner to get fit with and hold each other accountable.

You don't have to feel like you're going to faint to get results. Research has indicated that moderate levels of exercise are best for most people. This means breathing a little heavier than normal, but not so heavy that you're completely out of breath. Your body should feel warmer than when you started, but doesn't need to be overheated or super sweaty. You don't need to do weight training exercises that are rough on your joints. Simple movements that get your heart rate elevated will do the trick.

Don't be too tough on yourself. When it comes to fitness and our physiques, sometimes we don't feel like we're on par with others. If you don't have the body you want or you don't feel like you're accomplishing the goals you set for yourself, just know that that is normal. Most people are hard on themselves, and a lot of times it never feels like enough. Just begin, and trust that your body and brain *will* transform as you make fitness a part of your daily routine.

Something is better than nothing: If you're anything like me, there are some days where you just aren't feeling it. Maybe it was a long day and you're feeling tired, or your symptoms of anxiety or depression have drained you and working out is the last thing you want to do. That's perfectly fine! In fact, if that happens, take a day or night to yourself to do whatever it is that feels relaxing and comforting to you. For me, that's lying on the couch with my fiancée, watching a movie or show. You just have to make one small promise to yourself that tomorrow you will get a little bit of movement incorporated back into your life.

When you're under the gray cloud of depression or the paralyzing feeling of anxiety and you haven't exercised in a long time, it might feel like the biggest task in the world to get into fitness. Setting extravagant goals like completing a marathon or working out for an hour straight every morning at 5:00 a.m. could only lead to bigger disappointment if you fall short.

Doing just a few minutes of physical activity is better than nothing at all. Start with five or ten minutes. As an example, that could mean briskly walking from the front door of your apartment to the stop sign at the end of the street and back. The next time, try walking two stop signs down and back. Slowly you increase your distance. Make it fun, too! Bring a friend or significant other. The more you exercise, the more energy you'll have, and the more you'll want to do. The key is to shift your mentality to realize that something is better than nothing. You don't need to train like you're running a Spartan Race or CrossFit competition. You just need to get your body moving because it will pay dividends for your daily brain health.

Do activities you enjoy

Find a way to move your body that really feels good. That might be playing pick-up basketball at the rec center, running, dancing around your room to music, taking group cardio classes, rock climbing at a local park or on the rock wall at the gym, cycling, boxing, or power lifting. There truly is something for everyone. If one activity doesn't light you up, try something else.

Reward yourself

You're more likely to take action if there's a reward involved. Decide how you'll recognize your efforts. Maybe you treat yourself to a snack you love. Maybe you watch an extra episode of a favorite show. Maybe you give yourself an extra hour to scroll on Instagram. Whatever it is, make sure it's motivating enough to make you incorporate fitness into your life.

Virtual

There are so many virtual workout options now, including subscription-based models like Peloton. If you're strapped for cash, there are free options online, too. Follow a few fitness influencers on YouTube and Instagram and see if they have a schedule posted for the week. My fiancée and I take classes via Instagram Live, which is a great way to get exercise without leaving the house.

Getting out and moving your body should be fun, so find something to do that you enjoy. You don't have to spend hours in a gym or force yourself into long, monotonous workouts to get benefits from exercise. If you are currently in a state where your brain health is tough to balance due to feelings of depression or anxiety, take it easy on yourself. When you're dealing with these emotions, there are going to be days where you don't feel like doing much, and that's okay. Rather than looking at fitness as a checklist item that you have to do, look at it as a tool that can help boost your mood. You don't need to be the strongest, most in shape person at the gym. You just need to feel good after a workout, relieve some stress, and get endorphins flowing.

CHAPTER 17

USE RELAXATION TECHNIQUES

Five years ago, I accidently stumbled across an article that talked about meditation as a valuable practice. It explained that the highest-performing athletes and CEOs had adopted meditation as a valuable practice to optimize their job performance. I thought, "If CEOs and athletes are doing it, why not give it a shot?"

The challenge was that I had never meditated before. I thought, "How do I even do this?" It seemed so intimidating. You might be having the same thoughts. I was curious, though, so I started looking into it and ended up finding what was a little-known app at the time called Headspace. The beauty of this app was that a guy named Andy would do all the work for you. He would guide you through a ten-minute meditation, and all you had to do was show up, sit there, and do what he said. This sounded like something I could do! So I downloaded the app and told myself I would try out meditation first thing in the morning. That decision has changed my life forever—in all the best ways.

The next morning I ended up meditating for my very first time. During the process, Andy guided me the entire way. He had me start with my eyes open, taking deep inhales through my nose and exhaling through my mouth, releasing as much air as I possibly could. Next, he prompted me to gently close my eyes and get acquainted with my surroundings. I felt my body against the couch and attempted to listen to the sounds around me. He then asked me to do a body scan, from the top of my head down to my toes. After I had completed the body scan, he asked that I turn my attention to my breath. For this part, my job was "simple"—all I had to do was focus on my breath. Turns out it was not as simple as it sounded. I couldn't focus on it for more than five seconds before my mind started to wander. Every thirty seconds or so, he would gently guide me back to my breath. I struggled through this part until we finished the meditation session.

I only remember two takeaways from my first meditation session. The first, which is vivid, is that for ten minutes it felt like I was fighting my own mind to keep it focused on what Andy was asking me to do. When he asked me to focus on my breath, it felt like I could only string together one inhale and exhale before my mind started to wander. For the life of me, I couldn't keep focused. However, the second thing I remember is what kept me coming back.

Going into that first meditation, my heart was beating like a drum, my hands were shaking, my mind was racing, and I felt on edge, like I couldn't relax. After finishing that first meditation, I noticed a slight difference in my physiology and mood. My mind and body were more calm. I felt more focused. My pounding heart had subsided, and my racing thoughts had simmered down. I felt like I had more clarity. Most importantly, I felt relaxed.

I had no idea that this first experience with meditation would end up being the most important step I have ever taken to improve my life. Since 2015, I have rarely gone a day without taking ten minutes to be guided through a meditation. I've logged over seventeen thousand minutes of meditation. That's because what I've learned is that meditation is actually exercise for your brain that offers a wide variety of benefits. It gives me the much-needed relief from my anxiety and helps take the edge off. I don't just get peace for ten minutes, either; instead, sometimes I feel the benefits for the whole day.

You might be thinking to yourself, "Why should I care about relaxation techniques?! I can sleep when I'm dead. It's all about being productive, crushing goals and hitting the next benchmark." To you, I would say, "I respect that opinion. However, relaxation is a necessary part of being productive and cultivating great brain health." You will need a calm, well-trained, and rested mind to make important decisions in college and in your career moving forward.

What Is Meditation?

In the modern world, meditation has come to mean a lot of different things. Many people use the word *meditate* when they mean thinking or contemplating. Others use it to describe their prayer practice. For others, they believe it's about zoning out, having earth-shattering experiences, or even being able to control the mind. For me, I believed that meditation was a state I could reach in which my brain would be completely empty of thought. While my brain was empty of thought, I would enter into a new world where everything all of a sudden made sense. Basically, I thought meditation was something you did to achieve clarity on the meaning of life. As I have come to learn, I was slightly off in my beliefs. While meditation can help give you clarity about yourself and how your mind works, at its core it's about training the attention and being present.

According to Jon Kabat-Zinn, the founder of mindfulness-based stress reduction (MBSR), mindfulness is awareness that arises through paying attention, on purpose, in the present moment, nonjudgmentally. Meditation is not a part of any religion. It is a science, which means that the process of meditation follows a particular order, has specific principles, and produces results that can be verified and replicated.

When you meditate, you're dedicating a certain amount of time and effort to being as mindful as you can. This is done by choosing a meditation object, like your breath, and then paying attention to it. You follow your breath in and are aware that you're breathing in. You follow your breath out and are aware of your breath leaving your body. You will almost certainly notice that the mind naturally tends to wander. One moment you're paying attention to your breath, and the next you're thinking about a school assignment or replaying a scenario from a social interaction you had earlier that day. This is completely normal and okay. Rather than get frustrated and resist the natural tendency of the mind to wander or get caught up in thoughts, the goal is to gently refocus the attention on the breath.

Through this deliberate mindfulness, or paying attention on purpose, you can gain a host of medical benefits.

Health Benefits of Meditation

- Helps to manage stress, anxiety, and depression
- Increases immunity
- Lowers blood pressure
- Improves sleep
- Alleviates gastrointestinal difficulties
- Improves happiness and general well-being
- Enhances self-awareness
- Improves focus
- Increases kindness

Mindfulness improves brain health. Recently, psychotherapists have utilized mindfulness meditation as a key component in the treatment of depression, substance abuse, eating disorders, relationship conflicts, anxiety disorders, and obsessive-compulsive disorder.

Mindfulness improves well-being. It supports an attitude that finds gratitude in the simplicity of life. Being mindful helps you become fully engaged in whatever activity you are doing and helps strengthen resilience to deal with challenging moments. By deliberately focusing on the present moment, you take your mind out of the past or the future. This allows you to not get caught up in worrying about the future or ruminating on regrets. In turn, you become less worried about material success, which no one can ever get enough of, and instead develop deep connections with others.

Science Says about the Effectiveness of Meditation

- A 2014 review of 47 trials with 3,515 participants suggested that mindfulness meditation programs show moderate evidence of improving anxiety and depression.
- A 2012 review of 36 trials found that 25 of them reported better outcomes for symptoms of anxiety for groups that meditated compared to the control groups.

Getting Started on Your Own

You might be interested in trying out meditation but feel a degree of hesitation because you don't know where to start. It's normal to feel that way. When I first started meditating, I felt sort of awkward and unsure if I was even doing it right. For you, the process of getting started can be very simple. I would recommend you start by downloading a guided meditation app like Headspace or Calm. You can also download MyLife or look on YouTube for free guided meditations. The benefit of these apps or YouTube is that they provide all of the guidance you need to get started. Typically, the apps you have to pay for offer student discounts. Search your campuses website to see if they have any meditation clubs on campus you can join. This will help you find a community of like-minded individuals to grow with.

MEDITATION IS EXERCISE FOR YOUR BRAIN, THE SAME WAY THAT LIFTING WEIGHTS IS EXERCISE FOR YOUR MUSCLES.

With that being said, it might feel weird and awkward to start meditating. This is normal because you are developing a new skill, just like riding a bike. Meditation is exercise for your brain, the same way that lifting weights is exercise for your muscles. The more you do it, the more benefits you receive from it. It is the single most important thing I added to my daily life all those years ago. Below, I have laid out some basic tips for getting started on your meditation practice.

Don't try to do it without any guidance. Whether you choose to download a meditation app like Headspace or Calm or go to a meditation or yoga center, when you're starting out it's always best to start with guidance. For example, I use Headspace and have used it for the last four years. To this day I still opt to do guided meditations where Andy, the founder of the company, guides me through my breathing. It takes all of the pressure off of having to know what to do and allows me to focus on simply being present.

Don't think you need to meditate for absurdly long periods of time to reap the benefits. One of the biggest pushbacks I hear from people when I tell them to start meditating is that they don't have thirty minutes in their day to commit to just sitting. I don't blame them because I don't, either! Instead, I meditate each morning for ten minutes and then again in the evening to help myself relax and unwind. The great thing is that science has proven you only need ten minutes a day to start reaping the benefits.

Go with the flow. Don't get caught up in trying to stop your thoughts. It's impossible to stop your brain from thinking. Instead, gently bring your attention back to your breath and allow yourself to observe your inner thoughts, emotions, and bodily sensations without judging them as good and bad.

Find a place where you won't be distracted. When you first start out, it's important that you're somewhere peaceful and quiet. The place you choose doesn't need to be completely absent of noise, but you don't want a lot of foot traffic that could distract you or make you feel self-conscious if people see you.

Make sure you're comfortable. Make yourself comfortable but not so comfortable you doze off. I sometimes lie down on my couch, which is super cushiony, when I meditate. Other times I sit in a padded chair. The key here is to make it easier to relax.

Pick a time when you won't feel rushed. I meditate in the morning before work because I don't feel rushed. From my experience, it's a lot harder to carve out ten minutes to meditate once the momentum of the day gets started. So find a time that you know you can commit to, and then give it a shot.

Practice acceptance. You're learning a new skill. Developing new skills takes time. If you accept in advance that you won't be good at meditating in the beginning, you give yourself the space from judgment to grow in the practice.

Try and try again. You will be giving yourself the biggest gift of your life if you decide to start meditating regularly. Remember, if you miss your intended time to meditate, that's okay. Simply try again another time. If you feel like your mind is racing at first, that's okay too. Simply try again the next time. Each experience is unique, just like you.

Hopefully by this point I've convinced you to at least give meditation a shot. With a few taps on your phone, you can have an app like Headspace downloaded and be on your way to cultivating better brain health. To make sure you have some foundational principles when you start, I have included Jon Kabat-Zinn's seven attitudes of mindfulness below, in my own words.

7 Attitudes of Mindfulness

1. ***Non-judging:*** Being a witness of your own mind can be difficult. It requires that you become aware of judging and reacting to your inner and outer experiences. Take a step back to simply observe this happening.

2. ***Patience:*** The simple truth is that some things in life must unfold in their own time. Intentionally remind yourself not to be impatient because you feel tense, agitated, or frightened. Give yourself the space to have these experiences.

3. ***Beginner's Mind:*** An open mind allows you to be receptive to new possibilities. No two moments are the same, and each one contains its own unique experiences.

4. ***Trust:*** One of the most important life skills you can develop is a basic trust in yourself. It is more beneficial to trust your own intuition than to always look outside of yourself for guidance.

5. ***Non-Striving:*** The goal of meditation is to be yourself. The irony, according to Kabat-Zinn, is that you already are yourself. Striving to be different from what you are in the current moment puts the idea in your mind that you are NOT okay. The reality is that you are already enough. You are amazing as you are.

6. ***Acceptance:*** Recognize things for what they are in the present moment. If you feel anxious, accept that you're anxious. In our daily lives, we waste a lot of time resisting what's already fact. When we do this, we force a current situation into something we want it to be, which only creates more tension.

7. ***Letting go:*** The art of letting go can be difficult. As humans we tend to hold onto certain thoughts, feelings, and situations. There are other thoughts we try to avoid, to protect ourselves. Letting go is a way of letting things be, without grasping.

Other Relaxation Techniques

There are a host of other techniques and practices you can adopt to help cultivate greater peace of mind. At one point or another, I have tried all of these techniques and see the value in them. Every person is different, so some techniques you might prefer over others. That's okay. Go with what feels right, and trust your intuition. The goal is not to fill your life with more things to do, but instead to fill it with only the most essential things that help nurture and foster your brain health. Below are a few other techniques you can use to help build better brain health.

Yoga: This ancient Indian tradition is a system of physical, mental, and spiritual practices, performed to increase bodily and mental awareness and to develop the spirit. The benefits of yoga are seemingly endless, but here are a few well-known examples:

- Increases flexibility
- Increases muscle strength and tone
- Decreases stress levels
- Fewer symptoms of anxiety
- Reduces inflammation
- Improves quality of life

As a start, try incorporating yoga into your life once a week. From my personal experience, you'll notice a difference in random aches and pains in your body, as well as a general feeling of calm.

Sensory Deprivation Tank: Also known as an isolation tank or flotation tank, this technique is used for restricted environmental stimulation therapy. In normal people terms, this means you lay down in a tank of warm salt water with minimal sound, which allows your body to naturally relax. Based on my personal experience, I do feel more relaxed and calm after doing a session.

A study done in 2018 demonstrated that an hour-long session in a deprivation tank was able to significantly reduce the feelings of anxiety in the fifty participants who attended. In another study done in 2016, forty-six people with generalized anxiety disorder self-reported reduced symptoms of depression, less irritability, and less difficulty sleeping. Here are a few other benefits:

- Relieves tension headaches
- Improves sleep
- Reduces blood pressure
- Helps promote relaxation

- Speeds up muscle recovery
- Can enhance creativity
- Can help change bad habits
- Improves feelings of self-acceptance
- Improves relationships

The only challenge is that this relaxation technique can be a bit pricey. You'll more than likely need to drive off campus to find a business that has these tanks. If your school is located in a rural area, you might not be able to find one. With that being said, it is still worth trying out because it could be something you do on summer break or during a visit home.

Acupuncture: This is a form of alternative medicine and a key component in traditional Chinese medicine. In this practice, thin needles are inserted into the body at various places that have been identified over the years to help with all sorts of healing. Although there is a lot of conflicting scientific research on the efficacy of the technique, some claim that acupuncture:

- Reduces stress
- Reduces back pain, neck tension, and joint pain
- Relieves headaches
- Decreases eye strain
- Improves immune system functions
- Enhances mental clarity
- Increases energy
- Relieves digestive conditions

I've made acupuncture a weekly practice and have noticed improvements in neck and upper back tension. During the session, I melt into the table. Afterward, I leave deeply relaxed. A lot of times I end up taking a nap after a session because of how at peace I feel. Regardless of what the science says, I've noticed the benefits.

Massage: The goal behind a massage is to help alleviate tension in the body and mind. Bodywork from a trained massage therapist can bring relief for a lot of people. Massage can:

- Reduces stress, anxiety, and tension
- Calms the nervous system
- Relieves muscle cramps and spasms
- Promotes a sense of well-being and relaxation
- Reduces blood pressure
- Prevents injury
- Increases flexibility
- Assists in pain management
- Improves one's outlook on life

The mind and body are interconnected in ways that science is starting to prove. When the body feels better and relaxed, the brain tends to feel more relaxed as well. Take thirty or sixty minutes to treat yourself to a massage every now and again. Your mind and body will thank you.

You might be on the fence about starting to meditate because you don't think it will work for you or you won't be able to "do it right." I understand; I once held tightly to those same beliefs. The reality is this: at the core of meditating lies the belief that there is no perfect or right way to do it. It's more about showing up each day to connect with your breath and sit with your thoughts. You don't need to shut your mind off or resist thinking. Instead, meditation teaches you to allow thoughts to come and go like clouds in the sky while you connect with your breath.

All you need is a quiet spot to sit, ten minutes, a guided meditation, and your breath. Taking time to unplug and allow your mind to relax is one of the most important habits you can incorporate into your life, just like eating healthy and exercising. Meditation has improved my feelings of anxiety and stress, and I promise it can do the same for you.

CHAPTER 18

MONITOR YOUR SUBSTANCE USE AND TAKE THE RIGHT SUPPLEMENTS

As you continue to build out your brain health blueprint, you're going to want to become mindful of what substances you put in your body. This is because you need to understand the relationship between what you put in your body and how your brain reacts to those substances. For a lot of college students, part of their education while at school involves experimenting with alcohol, pot, pills, and other drugs. This was a part of the culture while I was in school and seems to still be the case when I speak to college students around the country.

In conjunction with the party culture at a lot of universities, coffee and stimulants are popular. It's not uncommon to hear about students drinking four or five coffees a day to give them energy to get through homework and studying. From personal experience, I can tell you that alcohol and caffeine do not always react well with an anxious and depressed brain. You, too, will want to consider the relationship you develop with these substances during your collegiate years.

Pass the Booze Bottle

Binge drinking can be a huge part of the college experience. You've probably heard or maybe even said, "I was so blacked out last night." Maybe you've taken pulls straight from the vodka bottle and crushed beer bongs with your friends. I've been there, too, in my experimentation phase, with heavy drinking while partying in college. It can feel exciting and cool to get super drunk with your friends. This behavior can become so commonplace that you don't even realize it's not healthy for you.

The reality is that drinking alcohol can impact your brain health in a couple major ways. For one, if you're struggling with stress, anxiety, or depression, alcohol can become a tool you use to cope with these emotions. For example, after a tough week of exams, you might want to blow off steam by drinking with your friends. You meet up with them, get super drunk off of cheap vodka, and wake up with your shoes still on. No doubt, it might've been a super fun night, but you could be starting to rely on alcohol as a way to relieve stress, meaning anytime you're feeling stressed, you reach for the booze to calm your nerves. You might not even be aware that you're using alcohol to help escape feelings of stress.

This same thought process applies to anxiety. You might drink large quantities of alcohol to help alleviate the anxiety you feel in social situations. Rather than learning to sit with that anxiety and be present with it, you numb yourself to it by drinking. For me, this was a tactic I started using before I even knew that what I was feeling was anxiety. As I've developed a relationship with my anxiety, I've learned that certain social situations make me feel anxious. In the past, I would've had a few drinks to make myself feel better, but now I intentionally sit with those feelings so I can build a resilience and not be dependent on a substance to make me feel better.

Depression and alcohol can have a very similar relationship. You might find yourself drinking to escape feelings of sadness. Rather than addressing what's going on internally, you numb yourself to the feelings through booze. While this might work temporarily, alcohol always wears off. Once its numbing effects are gone, you're left facing the feeling you were hiding from. To avoid facing that feeling, you might drink more, and more often, just to escape.

The cherry on top of the sundae of dependency is the hangover that will almost certainly follow the day after heavy drinking. For the depressed and anxious mind, alcohol leaving your system is like painkillers wearing off after a surgery: what's left are the feelings you were trying to numb out, except those feelings come back with a fury. Since alcohol is a depressant, your feelings of anxiety and depression will be worse than before you drank. Now, you'll spend an entire day feeling more anxious or depressed with a headache, upset stomach, and fatigue.

FOR THE DEPRESSED AND ANXIOUS MIND, ALCOHOL LEAVING YOUR SYSTEM IS LIKE PAINKILLERS WEARING OFF AFTER A SURGERY.

You, therefore, have to decide what type of relationship you want to have with alcohol as you learn to cope with anxiety and depression. My advice would be to limit how much booze you consume at the beginning of your brain health recovery process. Your brain is in a sensitive state right now, and it doesn't need a harmful substance in the mix. I'm not a clinician, but from my experience, if alcohol isn't going to help in the recovery process, then why bother with it? Once you're in a better brain space and those feelings of anxiety and depression are more manageable, then you can slowly introduce alcohol back into your life if that's something you decide you want.

Feeling Cracked Out

The feeling of caffeine kicking in is undeniably pleasant. You feel your brain waking up as the adrenal glands pump adrenaline through the body. Although this might feel great, caffeine can also have an adverse effect with anxiety. For the anxious brain, caffeine can be like throwing gasoline on a fire. It has the potential to intensify your feelings of anxiety; make you feel jittery; increase tension in your upper back, neck, and jaw; and make your mind race.

You need to decide what's best for you. As somebody who still utilizes caffeine, I can understand how you might believe you need it. However, if it's going to cause your anxiety to flare up and get worse, then it's worth weighing the costs and benefits. The middle ground for you could be switching to green tea, which has less caffeine. Regardless, it's important to protect your brain during this time and don't put anything in your body that could cause it harm.

Free Smoke, Free Smoke

As someone who was a pot smoker for years, I know that it can be a crutch to escape feelings of depression and anxiety. If marijuana is your choice of substance, I get it. What I want you to consider is whether or not you're getting high because you enjoy it or because you're trying to escape the brain health challenges you are facing. The answer to that question will tell you whether it should remain a part of your life or be removed. For me, that answer became very clear once I found myself craving it to escape from my feelings of anxiety. Once I stopped using it as a crutch, it opened up the door to lasting recovery by healthier coping strategies like meditation.

Popped a Molly I'm Sweatin'

Painkillers, Xanax, cocaine, and Molly can seem like appealing ways to enhance the party experience and feel a vibe. However, all of these can be addictive and dangerous, especially when you're mixing them with alcohol. Bottom line: do not take these recreationally if you're struggling with anxiety or depression. They have the potential to make you feel worse the day after taking them, as the drugs start wearing off.

Supplements to Consider

The supplements I'm about to recommend have been helpful to me. However, I am not a doctor, and you should *always consult with a doctor before taking anything.*

Fish oil: More and more studies are showing that inflammation in the brain can lead to increased feelings of anxiety and depression. Fish oil has been promoted as a natural anti-inflammatory that can improve brain health. For that reason, I take fish oil capsules twice daily to help with inflammation in the brain.

B12: I take B12 to help create natural energy in my body. For me, it works best when taken in powder form and mixed with water.

L-theanine: This component is naturally found in green tea. A double-blind 2019 study found a decrease in stress-related symptoms (i.e., depression, anxiety-trait, and sleep) and improvement in cognitive function after four weeks of L-theanine administration. This study concluded that L-theanine may be suitable for improving mental conditions in healthy populations. I have personally taken L-theanine on a daily basis for over three years and have noticed an improvement in my anxiety. I take it first thing in the morning via capsule form.

Turmeric: This spice has been used in Indian, Southeast Asian, and Middle Eastern cooking. It has inflammation-reducing properties. I typically take this supplement after lunch as a way to further reduce inflammation in my brain and body.

Ashwagandha: This supplement is a root found in India. It is used to help reduce feelings of stress and anxiety. I take it in capsule form as needed.

Magnesium: I use magnesium to induce relaxation and sleepiness in my mind and body an hour or so before bed. I take it in powder form and mix it with water. It works very well to help me calm down and relax.

Stress tea: There are a variety of teas that promote relaxation and reduce stress. I personally drink the cinnamon-flavored Stress Ease tea, made by Traditional Medicinals. From my personal experience, I've noticed that it helps me calm down at night, so I typically drink it an hour before bed as I start to wind down, to help me fall asleep.

Alcohol and caffeine are very common substances that are widely accepted and used in Western culture. As a young adult, you need to consider what type of relationship you want to develop with these substances based on how they react with your brain. They can have harmful effects on your brain and can make the situation worse if you are currently in the process of recovery. Be mindful of this as you are building out your brain health blueprint.

CHAPTER 19

BUILD A FOOLPROOF SUPPORT SYSTEM

I still remember the day I told my fiancée, with tears welling in my eyes, that I had been diagnosed with obsessive-compulsive disorder. She looked back at me and with a loving tone told me she loved me more now than before I told her. She didn't make me feel weird, weak, or different, but instead wanted to understand how she could help. This was the type of support I needed and the type of support I want to make sure you cultivate for yourself. On your road to recovery, it's important to ask for help. I've learned that your support system—the people you choose to surround yourself with—is an enormous part of how successful your recovery process is. Had I not had special people in my life supporting me on my journey, there is a chance I wouldn't be here. That might sound grim, but it's the truth. Support from others matters.

You're going to need loving, kind, and nonjudgmental support on your journey to sustained recovery. It's paramount that you build a team around you that can guide you every step of the way. By building out the right team, you'll not only guarantee your success in recovery, but also in other areas of your life. I've compiled a list of best practices to cultivate a support system, communicate with your support system, and provide support to others when they need you.

The Trap of Isolation

You might be feeling a pull to withdraw from other people. Maybe you just don't feel like talking to your friends or family. Perhaps it feels like it will take too much energy. You might believe people don't really like you. You might experience anxiety when you think about leaving your home or apartment to go interact with friends. Previously, you may have been a social person, but now you just want to hide away. These feelings and reactions are very common for people coping with depression and anxiety. There's a tendency to want to self-isolate. It's important that you don't fall into this trap because social isolation can lead to increased feelings of depression and anxiety.

An example of this could be wanting to spend an entire day in your room. You might have no desire to leave because you don't feel up to it, and so you stay there all day. That same day you receive text messages you choose not to respond to. Since you don't feel like talking to anyone, this behavior builds on itself. One day turns into two, which turns into a week. Before you know it, you've blown off all your friends and haven't left your house. This makes you feel even worse, and you start to beat yourself up worrying about what those people will think.

This example is something I've seen over and over from students that I coach. The ones dealing with depression and/or anxiety always tend to isolate themselves because of fear of judgment or lack of energy. As a result of that isolation, they feel lonely. That loneliness leads to more feelings of sadness because they feel cut off from their friends and family. This cycle continues until a change is made. You can begin to make a change by first becoming aware of when you start to withdraw. Once you start to notice that you're isolating yourself because of anxiety or depression, you can take the steps to combat isolation.

This can be done in small steps. You could start by texting a friend or family member and asking them, "What's up?" Start with something so easy that it takes no energy at all to reach out to them, and then build from there. Next, use that text conversation to invite a friend or family member to come hang out or take a walk with you. Even if you feel like you don't want to hang out with anyone, push yourself to maintain some social connection.

Your Support System

When building out your team, you should first consider people you can trust and who won't judge you. These people could include:

- Family members
- Friends
- Health care providers
- Co-workers
- Teachers
- Religious advisors
- Anyone else you trust
- Teammates

People in your support system play different roles. Here are a few roles you'll want to fill when building out your team.

The Rock: This should be your mom, dad, sibling, significant other, or someone you consider family. This person makes you feel supported and loved at all times. You can talk to them about whatever you're feeling or struggling with, and they're there to listen to you without judging. You feel safe with them.

The Genuine: As you build out your team, you want to consider a friend you can be your authentic, genuine self with. When you're with them, you don't have to hide anything or pretend you're someone else. Conversation flows naturally with this person. This is important because if you're already low on energy due to anxiety or depression, you don't want to have to expend more energy with a friend you can't be yourself around or connect with deeply.

The Pusher: This team member is critical to your recovery process because they will push you out of your comfort zone at times. For example, you might want to bail on an appointment with your therapist, but this friend or family member offers to go with you. They understand that you might not feel like it, but know it's best for you, so they push you.

The Exerciser: Another one of your support members should be your workout partner. Having a workout partner will ensure that you stay consistent with your fitness while having fun.

The Comedian: Laughter is a very important part of the recovery process and living a full life. One of your support members should be the funny one. Maybe you don't talk about anything deep with this person, but they bring joy into your life by making you laugh. At times in your journey, you'll need laughter to get through the challenging times, so having this person is important.

The Professional: Your licensed brain health professional should be the person you go to for medical advice. This might include numerous people, like a therapist, psychiatrist, general practitioner, etc., that you see at different times. This part of the team is critically important because they'll provide clinical steps you need to take to continue recovery. Don't be afraid to switch these individuals out for someone new if you don't feel like they're a good fit.

The Peer Supporter: A peer supporter is someone who's gone through what you're going through and is further along in the recovery process. They're important because they can provide "lived experience" support. This means that they can share what they've been through, what helped them improve, and help you find the right professional support. They'll also serve to remind you that recovery is possible, because they've been through what you've been through and have gotten better.

The Filter System

Everyone in your support system should share two characteristics: nonjudgmental and compassionate. Your team should be your biggest cheerleaders. They should never make you feel less than, stupid, weird, or embarrassed. They should want to see you win and get better.

It's okay to filter your support system so that it's truly supportive. If you feel hurt, upset, abused, judged, disrespected, or angry after hanging out with a certain family member or friend, you might need to limit your time with them. This can be difficult with family, as we don't get to choose our family members, but we do get to choose how we spend our time with them. If your friend is putting you down for dealing with anxiety or depression, then that's a sign you shouldn't hang out with them anymore. Your support system should be comprised of people who lift you up, not people who bring you down.

EVERYONE IN YOUR SUPPORT SYSTEM SHOULD SHARE TWO CHARACTERISTICS: NONJUDGMENTAL AND COMPASSIONATE.

Benefits of a Strong Support System

Social support can increase your brain health by:

- ***Alleviating stress:*** By having someone you trust to speak with about your internal struggles, you give yourself the opportunity to release bottled-up emotions. Never underestimate the power of a listening and loving ear from your support group. Feeling heard is one of the most important parts of recovery.

- ***Increasing self-confidence:*** Just being a part of a strong social support system that cares about you provides a feeling of being loved and important. This feeling of belonging is a critical aspect to human connection and fuels positive brain health.

- ***Decreasing feelings of loneliness:*** When you bond socially with another human, a hormone known as oxytocin is released into the body. This chemical is known to promote feelings of love, social bonding, and well-being. You were meant to connect with others because connection literally results in the release of positive feel-good chemicals in the brain.

Where You Can Find a Strong Social Support System

Whether you're new to a school or a senior in college, there's always an opportunity to make a friend to add to your support group. A good place to start to make friends is by getting involved in group activities that you enjoy.

- Join a fraternity or sorority
- Join an intramural league
- Find a meetup group that likes exploring new restaurants
- Find group fitness classes at your campus gym
- Enroll in classes that you are truly interested in and take time to meet others in those classes
- Join a club on campus (art, history, chess, science, etc.)

If Your Family Doesn't Understand

If you've confided in your family about brain health challenges and they don't understand what you're going through, it's important that you don't become discouraged. They might not be educated on brain health or have even a general understanding of what you might be feeling. Start by encouraging them to read a few articles on what you are coping with to help educate them. Typically, this helps provide context and clarity, so they know how best to support you.

If one of your family members is resistant to your emotions and downplays how you're feeling, try not to get upset. You cannot force someone into supporting you. This can be tough to comprehend with family, but by choosing to focus your energy with other people who do support you, you give yourself what your brain needs.

If Your Friend Doesn't Understand

If you confide in your friend about how you're feeling and they brush it off or downplay it, this might be a sign that they're not the best fit for your support group. Don't be discouraged or get upset with them. Instead, encourage them to read a few articles on your situation to learn more about it. If that helps, then great! If not, it might mean that you need to confide in other friends for support.

You've Got a Friend in Me

Want to confide in someone about what you're dealing with but not sure how? Here are some tips:

- **Remind yourself that brain health issues are common.** Like we've learned throughout this book, brain health issues affect millions of people. You're not weird or weak for experiencing these emotions. You're brave for opening up.

- **Make sure you feel very comfortable with the person you are opening up to.** I cannot emphasize this point enough. You might feel like you've really connected with someone, when in reality you've only known them for a few months. You have no idea how they'll react, so make sure you've thoroughly assessed someone's readiness to be your confidant before sharing with them.

- **Only share what feels comfortable at that moment.** It took me years to fully admit to my fiancée all of the symptoms I've experienced. Patience and comfort are key when opening up to someone. You're already stepping out of your comfort zone by sharing at all, so be gentle with yourself and divulge information as you see fit.

- **Pick a time and place to talk.** Early on I made the mistake of reaching out to a friend in the middle of a busy workday to try and confide in him about what I was going through. Right as I told him I was feeling depressed, he said he had to go and would call me back.

That call back never came, which left me feeling like he didn't care. Once you've identified the person you want to speak to, make sure you schedule uninterrupted time with them, so they can give you their full focus. Pick a place to talk where you'll feel comfortable sharing personal information. Your living room might be better than a busy coffee shop because it's quieter and more intimate.

- **Explain what your symptoms look and feel like to help the other person better understand.** For example, describe the tightness in your chest from anxiety or that you don't always have energy because of depression. Some detail can really help the other person empathize with what it feels like when you're struggling.
- **Let them know how they can support you.** Can they help you schedule doctor's appointments? Are there things you could do together to help you feel better? What's the best way for them to communicate with you? Loop them in.
- **Let them know whether what you're sharing is confidential.** This is pretty clear cut. If you want your friend to keep your conversation private, then make sure to clearly articulate that.

CHAPTER 20

MANAGE SOCIAL MEDIA

Few people are immune to the magnetic pull of social media these days. It can be tough not to spend hours scrolling, but for people dealing with depression and anxiety, the challenge of social media goes beyond that. If you're not intentional with how you use it, social media can have a major impact on your brain health. That's why you need to use your social media platforms in a way that serves you and doesn't make you feel worse. When you see your timeline filled with smiling faces, you might wonder if you're the only one who feels sad. You might follow influencers and celebrities who look like they have amazing lives and feel envy or shame. Comparing yourself to people on your feed can increase feelings of anxiety and depression. For this reason, you have to understand how social media is used today, how it impacts your brain health, and what you can do to protect your mental wellness.

IG Is about Impression Management

Looking back at my Instagram posts from 2016, there were pictures of me smiling, traveling to different cities, laughing with friends, and hanging out with my fiancée. To an outside observer, it looked like my life was great. However, my posts weren't a true reflection of the internal turmoil I was experiencing. I wanted people to think my life was awesome—partly because I wanted social validation, and partly because I desperately wanted to actually feel happy. I wanted to conceal the fact that in reality I was miserable, lost, and scared. The pictures I posted were nothing more than a facade, an attempt to brand myself as a guy who was going places and crushing goals. A guy who had it all figured out. In reality, I was battling anxiety, depression, and suicidal thoughts. I was uncertain about my future and how my life would turn out.

My posts were an example of a trend on social media today called *impression management*, essentially, how we filter information to shape our friends' perceptions of us. Oftentimes, this means crafting our social media persona to be confident, together, and popular. Unfortunately, this trend is heavily contributing to the uptick in anxiety, depression, and other emotional challenges. According to Dr. Janet Hibbs and Dr. Anthony Rostain, this phenomenon is causing many college students and young adults to feel incompetent and isolated. Impression management is lowering college students' sense of self-worth, which can contribute to feelings of hopelessness and inferiority.

Smoke and Mirrors

Approach your timeline with the understanding that what you see of the people you follow might not be the full truth. For example, you might follow someone on your campus who's in a sorority, looks like she has a ton of friends, goes to parties, and travels places during the summer. From your point of view, this person might look like she has a better life than you. She might have more followers than you and get more likes on her pictures.

What you might not realize is that behind the scenes she's deeply unhappy. She might be dealing with anxiety and depression. She might feel lonely and disconnected from her friends. Her whole sense of self-worth might be tied up in how people respond to her posts, and therefore she feels down when she doesn't get the kind of engagement she expects.

Most people aren't naturally good at being vulnerable. In a lot of cases, people aren't willing to disclose the more private and painful aspects of their lives: a tough breakup with a long-term girlfriend or boyfriend, arguments with your parents, getting fired from a job, dealing with a stressful semester, feeling lost, feeling alone, feeling sad, or coping with a falling-out with a close friend.

Most people on your timeline are only going to post pictures of themselves smiling, laughing, surrounded by friends, in different cities or countries, at parties, on rooftops overlooking the ocean, at the gym, or dressed in trendy clothes because it's what feels safe. Intentionally or unintentionally, we all want to appear successful and happy because that's what we all crave. We all want to be happy and successful in our lives all the time. Instagram and other platforms give you the opportunity to curate the appearance of a great life through the pictures you choose. Simply by posting a picture of yourself appearing to crush life, you're creating the impression that you're happy.

Here's the thing: Life is messy and imperfect. We're not always happy and we experience moments of failure or setbacks. That is just a part of the human experience. When we only show pictures of our "best lives" on IG or other social media platforms, we might be telling only half of the story. Even worse, we might not be telling the truth at all.

HERE'S THE THING: LIFE IS MESSY AND IMPERFECT.

When I posted on Instagram, I wanted to look like I had everything figured out, when in reality I was more lost than I had ever been in my entire life. To the outside world it probably looked like I had everything figured out—I know that because people would say that to me. They had believed my lie! Now, multiply that behavior and mindset across everyone you know, and you get millions of people "doing it for the gram." You get a society that on the surface level looks happy and successful all the time.

How do you think social media has impacted your happiness and sense of self-worth? If you're anything like me, it probably makes you feel worse. It might make you think, "Why can't I be happy like this person?" or "Why can't I be successful like so-and-so?" That thought process has the potential to deteriorate your self-worth and how you see yourself. It also pressures you to create a similarly immaculate—if dishonest—online presence.

Here's the good news: You can protect your mental wellness right now by changing your perspective. For starters, recognize that social media is a way for people to show their "best lives." The next time you scroll through your timeline, keep in mind that just because a friend of yours is constantly posting pictures of herself studying abroad in Italy for a semester doesn't translate to her being extremely happy all of the time. For all you know, she's extremely homesick and misses her friends from back home, but doesn't want to admit that because she wants to look cool traveling the world.

Start to cultivate acceptance for who you are as a person and where you are in life. The more you accept your strengths and weaknesses, and your likes and dislikes, the sooner you'll be able to scroll through your feed without feeling bad about yourself.

By making these two subtle shifts in perspective, you'll free yourself from the vicious cycle of impression management when you scroll social media. From my experience, you'll see a drastic improvement in your overall happiness and how you see yourself as a person.

Other Factors to Consider

The psychology of Instagram

Thanks to Instagram, we all get the opportunity to share pieces of our lives with the people who follow us. At a basic level, people post pictures to get likes, gain followers, and display their "best lives." What this has done is create a virtual popularity contest in which you get real-time feedback, quantifiable via likes, comments, and the number of followers you have.

With a few clicks of a button, you can quickly sum up where you fit in the popularity contest among your friends by seeing how many people follow you compared to your friends, who gets the most likes on their posts, and who appears to have the "best life." If you tie your self-worth and identity to your social media profiles, you open the door to feeling like you aren't enough or that your lifestyle isn't enough because of so-and-so on Instagram who appears to have a better life than you.

We do it for the likes

At one point or another, we've all fantasized about being well-known or famous. This is because it's human nature to want to be liked and respected. Whether we realize it or not, being liked and respected feels good because it means you're accepted by the group, which in evolutionary terms means you have a better chance for survival. Every single time someone likes your post, follows you on Instagram, or leaves a nice comment, your brain receives a small hit of dopamine. This chemical messenger is sent down a reward pathway, which makes you feel good and crave more. Dopamine is associated with food, exercise, love, sex, gambling, drugs . . . and now social media.

But chasing the dopamine hit that comes from likes, comments, and follows is a game we can't win. It will literally never be enough. According to a TED-Ed Best of Web video, social media addiction is just like an addiction to gambling or substances. The brain rewires itself to desire more likes, more follows, and more comments. When you post a picture of yourself and get positive feedback, it stimulates the brain to release dopamine, which again rewards that behavior and perpetuates that habit.

What happens when one of your posts flops? We've all been there. We post a picture with a caption we're proud of and wait for the likes to come pouring in . . . and then they don't. It doesn't feel good. It almost feels like you've been rejected and judged. This in and of itself might make you feel less than or embarrassed. Furthermore, as your expectations rise for the amount of social validation you receive per post, you also avoid posting about topics that won't lead to this kind of validation. This can be very limiting and might pressure you to reveal only the most "accepted" aspects of your life.

Does all this mean you should delete your account? Not necessarily. But as I mentioned earlier, it's important to be mindful when using social media, to ensure it serves you well.

Lack of in-person connection and disrupted sleep

According to Dr. Jean Twenge, between 2012 and 2018 there was an uptick in the number of teenagers and young adults experiencing feelings of anxiety and depression. Based on her research, she hypothesized that smartphones and social media were significantly contributing to these increases. From her perspective, there were two major drivers.

Number one: individuals in this age group were experiencing significantly less face-to-face interaction with each other and instead communicating through text and social media platforms. This caused them to feel disconnected on a deep emotional level. In-person human interaction is essential for all human-beings and has a significant impact on whether you feel connected or lonely and isolated. Even in situations where, proximity-wise, you are close to your friends, it's not uncommon to be on your phones scrolling through IG and responding to DMs. This has the potential to dilute your in-person interactions, which leads to less deeply connected friendships, ultimately impacting your brain health.

Number two: your age group isn't getting enough sleep because of time spent on your phones late at night when you should be sleeping. This is caused by the blue light your phone gives off, which tricks your brain into thinking it's daytime, so melatonin isn't released at the same rate. It's also because the content being consumed is psychologically stimulating, which doesn't allow your brain to wind down and relax naturally. This lack of sleep can lead to increased feelings of anxiety and depression. It can also make it more difficult to cope with the daily struggles of life because you have less energy.

Social Media Best Practices

1. ***Schedule time to use social media and limit your use.*** As with all things in life, on social media balance is critical to maintaining healthy habits. Deliberately set aside time to allow yourself to scroll through timelines, look through profiles, and surf the web. An example would be giving yourself 15–30 minutes to watch entertaining content on Instagram after two back-to-back classes. Equally important is scheduling time to not be on your phone. An example of this would be staying off your phone the hour before bed so that you can wind down and fall asleep peacefully.

2. ***Be mindful of when you decide to jump on social media.*** According to a study by Microsoft, the average human's attention span is now eight seconds. Be mindful of the habit of pulling out your phone and jumping on Instagram anytime there's a lull in conversation when with friends or family. Instead, focus on being present with your friends. Use your phone to schedule in-person hangouts, but once you're with those people, put your phone away. In my own personal life, this is something that I've had to work on because it's so easy to want to keep the mind occupied. However, it can make the people you're with feel like you're not engaged and interested in what they have to say. By cultivating in-person friends, you'll develop deeper relationships that make you feel good.

3. ***Get clear on what you're using social media for.*** Is your profile for personal or business use? Are you following someone for personal inspiration or because everyone else is? Are you on Instagram to look up pictures of a cool restaurant in your area, or did you just go down the rabbit hole for an hour? Be thoughtful with how you use social media. This will keep you balanced and ensure that you're using it the way you want to, without letting what other people are posting take over.

4. ***Use other people's posts as inspiration—not for comparison.*** It's human nature to compare yourself to others. Therefore it's extremely important to be aware of how someone's account makes you feel. Is it motivating you to be your best self or making you feel bad? Shift your mindset to use the accounts as inspiration to show up in your daily life and try your best.

5. ***Be picky with who you follow.*** If someone's posts continually make you feel bad about yourself, then it's time to unfollow them. There's no reason to expose yourself on a daily basis to an account that doesn't fill you up. It's that simple.

6. ***Be active, but think before you post.*** Sharing your own content feels better than just looking at others' posts. Just make sure you're thinking about what you're putting out into the world. Are you sending a positive message? Is your post showy and going to contribute to making others feel worse about themselves? Ask yourself, "How would this make me feel if I was on the other side viewing this content?" Posting content that helps others will make you feel better because you get the satisfaction of knowing that you contributed positively to someone's life.

7. ***Social media is a small snapshot of someone's life.*** You never know the whole picture. As we've discussed, we never truly know what someone is really going through. Understand that people would prefer to showcase the good rather than the bad. If you're in a dark spot, just remember that other people are probably experiencing the same thing, whether their posts indicate that or not.

8. ***Leave social media.*** You could take the plunge and delete your social media apps. This might seem unfathomable at first thought because you feel like you'll be out of the loop with your friends. After a few weeks, though, you'll notice that you no longer crave getting on those apps. Instead, it could be just what your brain needs to recalibrate. Even better, this detox might force you to pick up the phone and make a phone call or schedule time to hang out

with people in person, which will help build deeper, more meaningful relationships.

Social media can be an amazing tool to keep you connected with family and friends. However, it can become a source of stress, frustration, anxiety, and depression if not managed properly. Starting with a shift in perspective and following the simple health tips above, you can reap all the benefits of social media without the side effects of devaluing yourself or affecting your brain health in a negative way.

If you feel like social media is altering your mood and taking a break hasn't helped, consider reaching out to someone about it. Remember, seeking help is always the answer.

CHAPTER 21

SPEND TIME IN NATURE

Growing up, my family went on one big family vacation a year. In my younger years, the entire family would pack up the van and make the twelve-hour drive down to Florida. We would spend a week on the beach, hanging out and soaking up the sun. As we got older, though, my parents decided to shift to more outdoorsy trips. We started going to places out west like California, Wyoming, Montana, Idaho, Washington, and Colorado. On these trips we would do full-day hikes. The landscapes were beautiful and awe-inspiring. My sister and I had never seen anything like them. The issue? I hated to hike! So I complained. A lot.

I didn't see the point in trudging along on a dirt path through trees just to get to an end point and have to turn around. It felt pointless. I basically spent my teenage years griping and complaining every time we ended up on a hike that lasted for more than half an hour. This behavior, of course, didn't please my parents, but they continued to take us on these nature trips every year. They were determined to make sure we developed some type of appreciation for nature. But every year, I continued to voice my dissatisfaction. Then my symptoms of anxiety and depression kicked in.

In almost every setting—work, home, the grocery store, the gym, restaurants, and bars—I would feel overwhelmed. A constant undercurrent of overwhelm pulsed through my entire body. It felt like I could never relax. One day a friend asked me to go on a short hike with him through a local park. I wasn't excited to go because I didn't really think the terrain in that area was pretty, but I was miserable in my own skin as it was, so I figured getting out and moving my body couldn't hurt.

When I arrived at the park, my heart was beating faster than normal because of my anxiety, and I could feel cortisol pumping through my body. I was stressed and anxious: my new normal. We walked to the trailhead and started our hike through the dense forests of Raleigh. The trail winded us through trees. Later in the hike, we came across a stream. We had been hiking for a while, so we decided to take a break and sit on some rocks by the water. I distinctly remember getting deeply focused on the pattern of water currents running over the rocks. Then I noticed something else. My physiology had changed. My breath had slowed down drastically. My heart was no longer pounding. The tension in my jaw, neck, and chest had disappeared. My body felt calm. My mind was no longer racing with thoughts I couldn't stop. For the first time in a long time, I felt at peace.

If you already love immersing yourself in nature, then you're ahead of the curve. If you still need a little warming up, don't worry, you're not alone. There's been a demographic and geographic shift on a global scale. Humans officially became an urban species sometime in 2008. The United Nations reported that for the first time in history more humans live in urban areas than rural ones. The last US census reported that cities were growing at a faster rate than the suburbs for the first time in a hundred years.

Concrete jungles, car alarms, honking, and crowded streets are becoming our norm, and it's hurting our deep connection to the natural world. We've forgotten how psychologically restoring natural spaces are for our brains. But hope is not lost! Even if you've never stepped foot in nature and never had an interest in the outdoors, you can still reap the benefits of nature in "citified" settings. By shifting our perspective and the relationship we have with nature, we can all reconnect with the natural world and improve our overall mental well-being.

Nature Helps Calm Depression and Anxiety

The use of nature as a form of therapy for depression has gained interest from scientists, researchers, and doctors. Reconnecting with the natural world has been shown to ease symptoms of depression. According to evolutionary biologist Isabel Behncke, when we're depressed we become trapped in our own thoughts. We become prisoners of our own minds. But scientists have shown the correlation between improved symptoms of depression and time spent in nature. They believe this could be attributed to the feeling of awe that's generated inside of us when faced with natural landscapes. In his book *Lost Connections: Uncovering the Real Causes of Depression*, Johann Hari writes, "Faced with a natural landscape, you have a sense that you and your concerns are very small, and the world is very big—and that sensation can shrink the ego down to a manageable size."

Nature helps calm my anxiety because there's less stimuli. In a city, your brain is constantly on high-alert. When in nature, there's less to worry about. Your brain can naturally unwind and take in the scenery around you. The inherent tranquility of natural environments helps clear the mind of unnecessary worries. It reduces feelings of anger and tension created by stress. This promotes mindfulness and gratitude.

THE INHERENT TRANQUILITY OF NATURAL ENVIRONMENTS HELPS CLEAR THE MIND OF UNNECESSARY WORRIES.

Nature Reduces Stress

I'm willing to bet that while at school your life is pretty fast-paced and demanding. You wake up in the morning, rush to class, stay on campus for a good portion of the day, rush back for meals, study when you can find time, and hang out with friends. During this time, you're bombarded with texts, emails, phone calls, and notifications. All of this activity is flooding your nervous system, which can cause stress. So how can you unplug? This can be done by immersing yourself in nature.

Doing so creates a buffer from the connected world that allows your mind to naturally unwind and forces you to be present in the moment. Furthermore, research is emerging that shows that just looking at pictures of nature or simply hearing sounds of nature can help reduce stress. In Sweden, a study was carried out that tested the effects of viewing nature scenes on participants after they had been given a challenging math task. Each individual was given a stressful math task to complete. After the task had been completed, they were instructed to sit through fifteen minutes of either nature scenes, non-nature scenes, or a blank room. Participants who viewed nature scenes reported having the lowest levels of stress. This is just one example of how nature has the ability to reduce stress.

Nature Makes You Move

You might've heard this before, but sitting is the new smoking. Think about it, how much movement did you have today? Did you get up and go for a walk outside, or did you spend most of your day inside? For the most part, we live sedentary lifestyles in which hours of our lives are spent hunched over our laptops, scrolling through social media or playing video games with friends. I'm not saying these things are all bad. My laptop is how I wrote this book, how I facilitate virtual brain health workshops, and how I connect with coaching clients. But it's not the natural state we evolved from.

At one point in human history, our ancestors were nomads who traversed hundreds of miles a year, constantly on the move. Our bodies and brains became accustomed to that movement as a natural form of mood regulation. Being in nature encourages a healthy lifestyle that all humans need and crave deep down inside. The benefits of being in nature include increased energy levels and the release of feel-good chemicals that promote happiness and calm. The combination of exercise with the mood-boosting effects of nature can help address symptoms of depression and anxiety.

Natural Light Improves Sleep

Think about a night when you didn't sleep well. How was it the next day? Were you sharp and on your game, or did your brain seem foggy and slower than normal? Were you able to accomplish the goals you had set for yourself? More than likely no. This is because poor-quality sleep has been linked to moodiness, fatigue, irritability, and a depressed mood. It makes learning new concepts difficult and can even impact short-term memory. Sleeping problems have even been linked to increased symptoms of anxiety and depression. However, when you deliberately expose your body to natural light, it can help regulate your body's circadian rhythm. This inevitably improves your sleeping patterns, which leads to a clearer, kinder brain. By giving yourself a daily dose of sunlight, you allow your body to naturally regulate itself and ensure that you have a great night's sleep so you wake up feeling rejuvenated.

Nature Encourages Social Connection

As you learned in previous sections, human connection is something we all crave and need. It's the glue that holds societies together and ultimately what makes us feel like we belong. Human-to-human connection is vital for promoting feelings of belonging, which helps us to feel secure and socially bonded. Getting outside into nature forces you to disconnect from the virtual world and pour your energy into the people around you. Going hiking with another person is a great opportunity to talk about each other's lives—uninterrupted. It's an opportunity to be vulnerable with someone and not have to worry about them pulling out their phone while you're talking to them. It's also a great opportunity to experience the beauty of nature together. Completing a tough hike together has the potential to strengthen your bond. This can provide you with a deeper sense of belonging and reduce feelings of isolation and loneliness.

How Much Time Do You Need in Nature?

Not as much time as you might think! Researchers in Finland conducted an experiment measuring people's well-being in three different environments: urban streetscapes, busy city parks, and wilder forests. The Finnish Forest Research Institute team, led by Liisa Tyrvainen, discovered that people felt psychologically restored after just fifteen minutes of sitting outside in both the park and forest. Another study conducted by Gregory Bratman at Stanford University found that only fifty minutes of walking in a city park boosted people's moods. After ninety minutes, a walk yielded changes to the participants' brains that can protect against depression.

So What's Next?

All humans need time in nature to increase their feelings of mental well-being. It's time to find your local park and get outside!

A walk outside in nature is something I've never regretted, and it always improves my mood. Use Google, Google Maps, Apple Maps, or AllTrails to find local parks and hikes. Most parks and nature preserves are free. If there is a day-use fee, it's minimal, and the benefits are worth it. Take it from the guy who used to hate to hike. Nature is where it's at.

CONCLUSION

You're not alone, weird, or weak for struggling with anxiety or depression. You're not going crazy. It's okay to not be okay. You're a normal human being who's experiencing tough emotions, just like millions of other people. You don't need to feel guilty or ashamed of your feelings.

You are not mentally ill or mentally well. Instead, your brain health is a continuum that will fluctuate over the course of your life, based on a number of factors, like your genetics, daily challenges, and traumas. All of these factors can cause feelings of stress, anxiety, and depression.

Improving your brain health starts with seeking help from a licensed brain health professional and recognizing that you deserve to heal. Find a brain health professional who understands you and knows how to properly diagnose and treat you. You might need to see a few healthcare providers before finding the right fit—don't give up.

I didn't start my recovery process until I recognized I deserved to seek help and then began to search for the right brain health professional. It took a few tries, but I eventually found a psychologist who was able to properly diagnose me and start me on ERP talk therapy that worked specifically for OCD. If I had given up, I might not be here today. You, too, should continue to push. The right doctor is one phone call or text message away, so keep trying!

Remember, even as you begin to heal, there will still be challenging days, weeks, months, and even years. Despite being a brain health advocate, I still struggle with bouts of depression and severe anxiety. I have low days and weeks that really challenge me, when it's a struggle just to get by. You will experience those times as well. Whenever you find yourself experiencing these emotions, remind yourself that this too shall pass. Impermanence is one of the few truths in life. Everything is always changing, and that's just as true with your brain health.

EVEN AS YOU BEGIN TO HEAL, THERE WILL STILL BE CHALLENGING DAYS, WEEKS, MONTHS, AND EVEN YEARS.

If you do find yourself having suicidal thoughts, know that these are not thoughts that need to be acted on. The brain is a great liar when it's depressed. It can tell you that suicide is a viable option. It can trick you into believing that you'll feel this way forever. However, once you've begun to heal, more and more those gray clouds will lift, you'll start to feel happier, and you'll be grateful to be alive. Never make a permanent decision off of temporary emotions. I care about you, and you matter to this world.

Your long-term, sustained healing will be predicated on the mindsets you choose to adopt and the lifestyle you live. Consciously choosing to express your emotions instead of bottling them up will help you regulate how you feel. Just like steam must leave a heated teakettle, your emotions need a release. When you share what's going on with you with your trusted team, you diminish the power that anxiety and depression have over you.

In addition to cultivating vulnerability, forgive yourself for past mistakes and focus on what you can do moving forward. This can be done by setting meaningful goals that get you excited about life. These goals shouldn't be so big that they wear you out. The idea here is not to stress yourself out, but to get you excited. As you graduate from college and move into the working world, know now that having the goal of finding meaningful work could increase feelings of stress, anxiety, and depression, in part because those types of jobs are very hard to come by. Plus, there's no guarantee that meaningful work will make you infinitely happier. Instead, your job might serve as the tool you need to pay bills and do things you enjoy. That's completely fine.

Lastly, as you build out your brain health blueprint, prioritize sleep, meditation, and physical activity as part of your daily routine. Schedule your entire day around when you want to go to sleep and when you want to get up. If you can swing it, try to schedule your classes later in the morning so you have time to sleep in, and get as much sleep as possible. When it comes to meditation, you only need ten minutes of it each day to exercise your mind and decrease feelings of stress, anxiety, and depression. Give yourself the gift of meditation. I promise it's worth it.

Very soon, one of these days, after you've sought professional help, opened up about your feelings, received a diagnosis, been put on a treatment plan, and started to live a healthy lifestyle, you'll wake up and notice that your brain feels better. Then, after a little more time, you'll notice an improvement again. Eventually, you'll wake up and notice a complete shift in how you feel. Your anxiety or depression will have lifted, and you'll feel like yourself again. It won't be quite the same you because you will have grown and evolved from this experience. You will have become a better version of yourself, and I can't wait to meet that person.

The time is now. You're young, and you have your whole life ahead of you. Take your brain health seriously, and don't delay joy. I'll leave you with this quote by Christine Caine: "Sometimes when you're in a dark place it feels like you've been buried alive. But perhaps, you've just been planted and now is your time to bloom."

RESOURCES AND WAYS TO GET INVOLVED

Crisis Hotlines and Chat

If you're in crisis, don't wait to reach out to a crisis line. There are a variety of hotlines you can contact right now, including:

- The Suicide Prevention Lifeline: **1-800-273-8255**. They have an option for individuals who are deaf or hard of hearing. You can also utilize their website to find psychologists in your local area.
- The Crisis Text Line: text **HOME** to **741741**.
- The NAMI helpline: **1-800-950-6264**. This line is staffed by volunteers who have mental health conditions, who provide information and resource referrals.
- SAMHSA's National Helpline: **1-800-662-4357**. They don't provide counseling, but will transfer you to appropriate intake centers in your state.
- The Disaster Distress Helpline: text **TalkWithUs** to **66745**.
- The LGBT National Help Center Hotline: **1-888-843-4564**. Volunteers identify as being on the LGBTQ spectrum and are trained specifically to support members of the LGTQIA community.

- The National Domestic Violence Hotline: Call **1-800-799-7233**. If you're unable to safely call, you can log onto thehotline.org or text **LOVEIS** to **1-866-331-9474**.

Related Organizations

The Peace of Mind Foundation: The Peace of Mind Foundation is a nonprofit dedicated to providing resources and support to those impacted by obsessive-compulsive disorder (OCD) and related disorders. Through education, research, support, and advocacy, the foundation is determined to help individuals worldwide access the information and tools they need to manage their OCD: peaceofmind.com.

One Mind: One Mind is a patient-centric brain health nonprofit organization that focuses on healing the lives of people impacted by brain illness and injury. Shari and Garen Staglin launched One Mind in 1995 as a way to bridge the gaps they saw in mental health patient support after their son Brandon was diagnosed with schizophrenia. Ever since, One Mind has become a leading mental health nonprofit that works to unite brain health professionals, business leaders, and politicians to improve brain health research and treatment: onemind.org.

National Alliance on Mental Illness: NAMI is the nation's largest grassroots mental health organization dedicated to building better lives for the millions of Americans affected by mental illness: nami.org.

Mental Health America: MHA is the nation's leading community-based nonprofit dedicated to addressing the needs of those living with mental health challenges: mhanational.org.

National Suicide Prevention Lifeline: The National Suicide Prevention Lifeline is a national network of local crisis centers that provides free and confidential emotional support to people in suicidal crisis or emotional distress 24/7. They're committed to improving crisis services and advancing suicide prevention by empowering individuals, advancing professional best practices, and building awareness: suicidepreventionlifeline.org.

Additional Resources

TherapyForBlackMen.org: TherapyForBlackMen.org is an organization dedicated to helping men of color find the right therapist. Using the directory, men of color can search for therapists based on location and specialization. In addition, they offer a wide range of resources to help men of color on their brain health journey: therapyforblackmen.org.

The National Alliance for Hispanic Health: The National Alliance for Hispanic Health was founded in 1973 in Los Angeles to provide mental health resources for the Hispanic community. They are one of the premier science-based organizations focused on better health for all. They provide services for more than 15 million Hispanics throughout the US every year: healthyamericas.org.

Therapy for Latinx: Therapy for Latinx utilizes technology to provide national mental health resources for the Latinx community. They can help connect you with a licensed therapist who speaks Spanish and understands the challenge you face culturally: therapyforlatinx.com.

Anxiety and Depression Association of America: ADAA is an international nonprofit organization committed to the treatment and cure of anxiety, depression, OCD, PTSD, and co-occurring disorders. They are a leader in mental health education, training, and research. ADAA provides evidence-based information and free resources on their website: adaa.org.

Therapy for Black Girls: Therapy for Black Girls is an online space committed to promoting the mental wellness of black women and girls. In addition, you can find therapists in your local area on their website: therapyforblackgirls.com.

The Association of Black Psychologists: The Association of Black Psychologists is a therapist resource directory comprised of members who own and operate their own private practices or are employed as therapists. You can use this directory to search for therapists in your state: abpsi.org.

Therapy for Queer People of Color: QPoC is a mental health network based out of Atlanta, Georgia. They offer services to help support your gender identity. In addition, they offer CBT, cognitive processing therapy, and cognitive behavioral couples therapy: therapyforqpoc.com.

Therapy for Asian Americans and Pacific Islanders: TAAPI is dedicated to assisting people in Asian American and Pacific Islander communities get connected with a therapist who understands their specific needs. Each therapy session offers you a private space to discuss what is most important to you: therapyforasians.com.

LGBTQ+ Community on Talkspace: If you identify as LGBTQ and are struggling with your brain health, Talkspace offers support from therapists who specialize in LGBTQ+ issues: talkspace.com.

Gaylesta: The Psychotherapist Association for Gender and Sexual Diversity is the largest group of individuals focused on LGBTQ mental health. They offer resources for those seeking therapy and will help match you with a therapist who understands your unique challenges: gaylesta.org.

Suggested Reading

- *Lost Connections: Uncovering the Real Causes of Depression—and the Unexpected Solutions* by Johann Hari
- *Cognitive Behavioral Therapy Made Simple: 10 Strategies for Managing Anxiety, Depression, Anger, Panic, and Worry* by Seth J. Gillihan PhD
- *Dare: The New Way to End Anxiety and Stop Panic Attacks* by Barry McDonagh

- *The Art of Happiness: A Handbook for Living* by His Holiness the 14th Dalai Lama
- *10% Happier: How I Tamed the Voice in My Head, Reduced Stress Without Losing My Edge, and Found Self-help That Actually Works* by Dan Harris
- *Black Pain: It Just Looks Like We're Not Hurting* by Terrie M. Williams
- *A Common Struggle: A Personal Journey through the Past and Future of Mental Illness and Addiction* by Patrick J. Kennedy
- *The Stressed Years of Their Lives: Helping Your Kid Survive and Thrive During Their College Years* by Dr. B. Janet Hibbs and Anthony L. Rostain
- *Overcoming Obsessive Thoughts: How To Gain Control of Your OCD* by Christine Purdon and David A. Clark
- *Shook One: Anxiety Playing Tricks on Me* by Charlamagne Tha God
- *The Unapologetic Guide to Black Mental Health: Navigate an Unequal System, Learn Tools for Emotional Wellness, and Get the Help You Deserve* by Rheeda Walker PhD

How Can I Get Involved?

I'm glad you asked! There are many different ways to get involved in the movement to normalize mental health and advance the community, so that more people can live free and happy.

Start by seeking help from a qualified mental health professional if you're struggling with any brain health challenges. By seeking help and beginning your journey to recovery, you'll demonstrate to the people in your social circle that it's normal and okay to seek help for their challenges. That normalization will have a ripple effect across society. BE the CHANGE by leading by example.

Consider donating to the mental health nonprofits that are tirelessly working to #smashthestigma associated with mental health, provide resources and support for struggling individuals, and find better treatments and cures. There are many organizations to choose from, so pick the one that resonates with you the most. I partner with One Mind and the Peace of Mind Foundation.

Volunteer and get involved via advocacy with nonprofits like the National Alliance on Mental Illness or Mental Health America. On their websites, you can find various ways to help. There are options to participate in a mental health awareness walk, attend a national convention, or even share your story. They are always in need of more loving and caring people who want to help move the cause forward.

Fourth, vote for politicians and bills that make mental healthcare more affordable and accessible to all people in the United States and worldwide. To see who supports the advancement of mental healthcare in America, you can visit: https://www.nami.org/Advocacy.

Share your story of recovery with everyone you know (if you feel comfortable). Stories have the power to move people to action. They change the way we perceive different situations. Your story is important, so share it.

Finally, lend a loving, listening ear every chance you get. Whether it's a friend, family member, or stranger sharing their mental health journey with you, I hope you take the time to listen. Allowing others to comfortably and safely express where they are in life opens up the door to recovery.

#YoureNotAlone

If you believe in the message of this book, please post a picture of you with the book on Instagram or Facebook with the hashtag #YoureNotAlone. If you feel comfortable, you can even share your brain health story if you want! You never know who needs to hear it. You're a part of a movement that is smashing the stigma of mental health and helping other people feel hope. Thank you, and I wish you the best on your journey!

REFERENCES

American College Health Association, *American College Health Association-National College Health Assessment II: Reference Group Executive Summary Fall 2018*. Silver Spring, MD: 2018.

American Psychological Association and American Institute of Stress. "What Is Stress?" Updated July 8, 2014, https://www.stress.org/daily-life.

Belluz, Julia, and Eliza Barclay. "The Growth of Yoga and Meditation in the US Since 2012 Is Remarkable." *Vox*, November 8, 2018. www.vox.com/2018/11/8/18073422/yoga-meditation-apps-health-anxiety-cdc.

Bennike, Ida H., Anders Wieghorst, and Ulrich Kirk. "Online-Based Mindfulness Training Reduces Behavioral Markers of Mind Wandering." *Journal of Cognitive Enhancement* 1 (June 2017): 172–181. https://link.springer.com/article/10.1007/s41465-017-0020-9.

BestColleges. "The Top Mental Health Challenges Facing Students." Updated May 6, 2020, www.bestcolleges.com/resources/top-5-mental-health-problems-facing-college-students/.

Brainworks. "What Are Brainwaves?" Undated, https://brainworksneurotherapy.com/what-are-brainwaves.

Bratman, Gregory N., J. Paul Hamilton, Kevin S. Hahn, Gretchen C. Daily, and James J. Gross. "Nature Experience Reduces Rumination and Subgenual Prefrontal Cortex Activation." *PNAS* 112, no. 28 (July 14, 2015): 8567–72. www.pnas.org/content/112/28/8567.

Breus, Michael. "5 Things To Know About Sleep And Inflammation." Updated January 1, 2019, https://thesleepdoctor.com/2019/01/01/5-things-to-know-about-sleep-and-inflammation/.

Brown, Brené. *Daring Greatly: How the Courage to Be Vulnerable Transforms the Way We Live, Love, Parent, and Lead*. New York: Penguin Random House, 2017.

Cafasso, Jacquelyn. "Traumatic Events." Healthline. Updated July 8, 2017, https://www.healthline.com/health/traumatic-events.

Canadian Mental Health Association. "Working with Your Doctor for Mental Illnesses." Here to Help. Last updated 2011. Undated. www.heretohelp.bc.ca/infosheet/working-with-your-doctor-for-mental-illnesses.

Casper, Rosanna. "How to Ditch the Victim Mentality and Become More Empowered." Lifehacker. Updated October 22, 2015, https://lifehacker.com/how-you-can-ditch-the-victim-mentality-and-become-empow-1738077671.

Chandrasekhar, K, Jyoti Kapoor, and Sridhar Anishetty. "A Prospective, Randomized Double-Blind, Placebo-Controlled Study of Safety and Efficacy of a High-Concentration Full-Spectrum Extract of Ashwagandha Root in Reducing Stress and Anxiety in Adults." *Indian Journal of Psychological Medicine* 34, no. 3 (July 2012): 255–62. www.ncbi.nlm.nih.gov/pmc/articles/PMC3573577/.

Cigna. "Loneliness Is at Epidemic Levels in America." Updated 2018, https://www.cigna.com/about-us/newsroom/studies-and-reports/combatting-loneliness/.

Corrigan, Patrick W., and Amy C. Watson. "Understanding the Impact of Stigma on People with Mental Illness." *World Psychiatry* 1, no. 1 (February 2002): 16–20. www.ncbi.nlm.nih.gov/pmc/articles/PMC1489832/.

DDS SafetyNet. "Social Support Systems and Maintaining Mental Health." Undated. www.ddssafety.net/sites/default/files /attachments/10-06-11/FASocialSupportSystem.pdf.

Ghanean, Heila, Amanda K. Centi, and Sidney H. Kennedy. "Fatigue in Patients with Major

Depressive Disorder: Prevalence, Burden and Pharmacological Approaches to Management." *CNS Drugs* 32, no. 1 (January 30, 2018): 65–74. https://link.springer.com/article/10.1007 %2Fs40263-018-0490-z.

Giliberti, Mary. "The Importance of Getting the Right Treatment for You," NAMI, 2017. www.nami.org/Blogs/From-the-CEO /October-2017/The-Importance-of-Getting-the-Right -Treatment-for.

Gillihan, Seth J. *Cognitive Behavioral Therapy Made Simple: 10 Strategies for Managing Anxiety, Depression, Anger, Panic, and Worry*. Emeryville, CA: Althea Press, 2018.

Glasofer, Deborah R., PhD. "Acceptance and Commitment Therapy (ACT) for GAD." Verywell Mind, February 29, 2020, www.verywellmind.com/acceptance-commitment-therapy-gad -1393175.

Goertemiller Carrigan, Catherine, and Denis J. Lynch. "Managing Suicide Attempts: Guidelines for the Primary Care Physician." *Primary Care Companion to the Journal of Clinical Psychiatry* 5, no. 4 (August 2003): 169–74. www.ncbi.nlm.nih.gov/pmc /articles/PMC419387/.

Gross, Terry. "College Students (And Their Parents) Face a Campus Mental Health 'Epidemic.'" *Fresh Air*, NPR, May 28, 2019. www .npr.org/sections/health-shots/2019/05/28/727509438/college -students-and-their-parents-face-a-campus-mental-health -epidemic.

Hari, Johann. *Lost Connections: Why You're Depressed and How to Find Hope*. London: Bloomsbury, 2018.

Harris, Dan. *10% Happier: How I Tamed the Voice in My Head, Reduced Stress without Losing My Edge, and Found Self-Help That Actually Works, a True Story*. New York, NY: HarperCollins, 2019.

Harris, Russell. "Embracing Your Demons: An Overview of Acceptance and Commitment Therapy." Psychotherapy .net. Updated 2020, https://www.psychotherapy.net/article /Acceptance-and-Commitment-Therapy-ACT.

Harvard Health. "Benefits of Mindfulness." HelpGuide.org. Updated 2020, www.helpguide.org/harvard/benefits-of-mindfulness.htm.

Harvard Health Publishing. "Exercise Is an All-Natural Treatment to Fight Depression." Harvard Health. Updated March 25, 2019, www.health.harvard.edu/mind-and-mood/exercise-is-an -all-natural-treatment-to-fight-depression.

Headspace. "The Science-Backed Benefits of Meditation." Updated 2020, https://www.headspace.com/science/meditation-benefits.

———"Learn How to Handle Tough Times to Help Your Headspace." Updated July 23, 2018, https://headspace .org.au/young-people/learn-how-to-handle-tough-times -to-help-your-headspace/.

———"Tips To Keep Good Mental Health." Updated October 1, 2018. https://headspace.org.au/young-people/tips-for-a -healthy-headspace/.

Health Research Funding. "21 Interesting Depersonalization Disorder Statistics." Updated January 13, 2015. https://healthresearch funding.org/21-interesting-depersonalization-disorder-statistics/.

Hibbs, Dr. B. Janet, and Anthony L. Rostain. *The Stressed Years of Their Lives: Helping Your Kid Survive and Thrive during Their College Years*. New York: St. Martin's Press, 2019.

Hidese, Shinsuke, Shintaro Ogawa, Miho Ota, Ikki Ishida, Zenta Yasukawa, Makoto Ozeki, and Hiroshi Kunugi. "Effects of L-Theanine Administration on Stress-Related Symptoms and Cognitive Functions in Healthy Adults: A Randomized

Controlled Trial." *Nutrients* 11, no. 10 (October 3, 2019): 2362. https://www.ncbi.nlm.nih.gov/pmc/articles/PMC6836118/.

Kabat-Zinn, Jon. *Full Catastrophe Living: Using the Wisdom of Your Body and Mind to Face Stress, Pain, and Illness*. New York: Bantam Books, 2013.

Knutson, Kristen L., and Eve Van Cauter. "Associations between Sleep Loss and Increased Risk of Obesity and Diabetes." *Annals of the New York Academy of Sciences* 1129 (2008): 287–304. www.ncbi.nlm.nih.gov/pmc/articles/PMC4394987/.

Levy, Jillian. "What Are Endorphins? (Plus, Hacks to Trick Your Body into Manufacturing More of These Feel-Good Chemicals.)" Dr. Axe. Updated June 19, 2017, https://draxe.com/health/what-are-endorphins/.

Lyons, Gila. "This Common Anxiety Symptom Makes Me Feel Like Reality Is Slipping Away." Healthline. Updated June 26, 2018, https://www.healthline.com/health/mental-health/derealization-anxiety-symptom-makes-reality-melt-away.

Manson, Mark. *The Subtle Art of Not Giving a F*ck: A Counterintuitive Approach to Living a Good Life*. New York: HarperCollins, 2019.

Mayo Foundation for Medical Education and Research. "Job Burnout: How to Spot It and Take Actions." Updated November 21, 2018, https://www.mayoclinic.org/healthy-lifestyle/adult-health/in-depth/burnout/art-20046642.

Mayo Foundation for Medical Education and Research. "Mental Health: Overcoming the Stigma of Mental Illness." Updated May 24, 2017, www.mayoclinic.org/diseases-conditions/mental-illness/in-depth/mental-health/art-20046477.

McDonagh, Barry. *Dare: The New Way to End Anxiety and Stop Panic Attacks*. Beaverton, OR: BMD Publishing, 2015.

McSpadden, Kevin. "You Now Have a Shorter Attention Span Than a Goldfish." *Time*, May 14, 2015. https://time.com/3858309/attention-spans-goldfish/.

Mental Health America, *The State of Mental Health in America*, 2020. www.mhanational.org/issues/state-mental-health-america.

Miller, John J., Ken Fletcher, and Jon Kabat-Zinn. "Three-Year Follow-up and Clinical Implications of a Mindfulness Meditation-Based Stress Reduction Intervention in the Treatment of Anxiety Disorders." *General Hospital Psychiatry* 17, no. 3 (May 1995): 192–200. www.sciencedirect.com/science/article/abs/pii/016383439500025M.

Mind.org. "Cognitive Behavioural Therapy." Undated. www.mind.org.uk/information-support/drugs-and-treatments/cognitive-behavioural-therapy-cbt/about-cbt/.

Mindworks. "Health Benefits of Meditation." Undated, https://mindworks.org/blog/health-benefits-of-meditation/.

Mindworks. "Meditation Definition: What Is Meditation? Take Charge of the Mind." Undated. https://mindworks.org/blog/meditation-definition/.

Mitchell, Caroline, Brian McMillan, and Teresa Hagan. "Mental Health Help-Seeking Behaviours in Young Adults." *The British Journal of General Practice* 67, no. 654 (January 2017): 8–9. www.ncbi.nlm.nih.gov/pmc/articles/PMC5198588/.

Mitchell, Sharon. "Emerging Trends in College Student Mental Health." Leadership Exchange. Updated 2019, www.leadershipexchange-digital.com/leadershipexchange/2019winter/MobilePagedArticle.action?articleId=1451365#articleId1451365.

Mohan, Pavithra. "Why Finding 'Meaningful Work' Is Overrated." *Fast Company*, April 8, 2019. www.fastcompany.com/90329998/why-finding-meaningful-work-is-overrated.

NAMI. *Mental Health By the Numbers*. September 2019. www.nami.org/mhstats.

National Center for Complementary and Integrative Health. "Meditation." US Department of Health and Human Services, April 2016. www.nccih.nih.gov.

National Sleep Foundation. "Healthy Sleep Tips." Updated July 30, 2020, www.sleepfoundation.org/articles/healthy-sleep-tips.

———"Relaxation Exercises for Falling Asleep." Updated July 28, 2020, https://www.sleepfoundation.org/shift-work-disorder/shift-work-you/relaxation-exercises-falling-asleep.

O'Grady, Dennis. "10 Introductory Questions Therapists Commonly Ask." PsychCentral. Updated July 8, 2018, https://psychcentral.com/blog/10-introductory-questions-therapists-commonly-ask/.

Pathak, Neha. "How Sleep Affects Your Health." WebMD, February 21, 2020. https://www.webmd.com/sleep-disorders/poor-sleep-affects-health.

Robinson, Lawrence, Jeanne Segal, and Melinda Smith. "The Mental Health Benefits of Exercise." HelpGuide.org. Updated June 2019, https://www.helpguide.org/articles/healthy-living/the-mental-health-benefits-of-exercise.htm.

Sack, David. "5 Important Reasons to Stop Ignoring Your Mental Health." *HuffPost*, March 5, 2014. www.huffpost.com/entry/healthy-living-news_b_4494887.

Santi, Jenny. "The Science Behind the Power of Giving." LiveScience. Updated December 1, 2015, www.livescience.com/52936-need-to-give-boosted-by-brain-science-and-evolution.html.

Santos-Longhurst, Adrienne. "Everything You Need to Know about Sensory Deprivation Tank Therapy." Healthline. Updated April 13, 2020, www.healthline.com/health/sensory-deprivation-tank.

Seppälä, Emma. "20 Scientific Reasons to Start Meditating Today." *Psychology Today*, September 11, 2013. www.psychologytoday.com/us/blog/feeling-it/201309/20-scientific-reasons-start-meditating-today.

Smith, Melinda, Lawrence Robinson, and Jeanne Segal. "Helping Someone with Depression." HelpGuide.org. Updated October 2019, www.helpguide.org/articles/depression/helping-someone-with-depression.htm.

Stanborough, Rebecca Joy. "Benefits of Reading Books: How It Can Positively Affect Your Life." Healthline. Updated October 15, 2019, www.healthline.com/health/benefits-of-reading-books.

Susman, David. "8 Reasons Why People Don't Get Treatment for Mental Illness." David Susman PhD. Updated June 2, 2017, http://davidsusman.com/2015/06/11/8-reasons-why-people-dont-get-mental-health-treatment/.

TEDEd. "5 Ways Social Media Is Changing Your Brain." Updated 2019, https://ed.ted.com/best_of_web/qQzsdX2Y.

Thompson, Andrew. "10 Ways Nature Benefits Your Mental Health." Go Green. Updated 2017, www.gogreen.org/blog/10-ways-nature-benefits-your-mental-health.

Tlalka, Stephany. "Meditation Is the Fastest Growing Health Trend in America." *Mindful*, December 11, 2018. https://www.mindful.org/meditation-is-the-fastest-growing-health-trend-in-america/.

Trauma Recovery. "Phases of Trauma Recovery." Updated 2013, https://trauma-recovery.ca/recovery/phases-of-trauma-recovery/.

Twenge, Jean. "Mental Health Issues Increased Significantly in Young Adults Over Last Decade." American Psychological Association. Updated March 14, 2019, www.apa.org/news/press/releases/2019/03/mental-health-adults.

US Centers for Medicare & Medicaid Services. "The Mental Health Parity and Addiction Equity Act (MHPAEA)." CMS, 2020. www.cms.gov/CCIIO/Programs-and-Initiatives/Other-Insurance-Protections/mhpaea_factsheet.

Wells, Katie. "Ecotherapy: The Health Benefits of Nature." Wellness Mama. Updated May 22, 2020, https://wellnessmama.com/56086/nature-health-benefits/.

Williams, Florence. "How Just 15 Minutes of Nature Can Make You Happier." *Time*, February 7, 2017. https://time.com/4662650/nature-happiness-stress/.

World Health Organization. *Mental Disorders*. World Health Organization, 2020. www.who.int/en/news-room/fact-sheets/detail/mental-disorders.

ACKNOWLEDGMENTS

First of all, I want to thank my soon-to-be wife, Katelyn (soon-to-be Westerbeck) Coburn. You have been there with me from the very onset of my symptoms. I still remember that rainy day in Raleigh, NC, when I told you I had been diagnosed with a chronic brain disorder known as OCD. I cried and you listened. After I was finished, you looked back at me and told me, "I love you more now than I did before you told me." Those kind words brought me more comfort than you'll ever know. They lifted my spirits and helped me to push forward on my path to recovery. Five years later and you are still my source of strength and inspiration. You push me when necessary, but are gentle and loving, too. You are without a doubt the love of my life. I love you.

I want to thank my parents and sister. To my mother, you received the very first distraught phone calls as I grappled with what was unfolding in my brain. You never once wavered in your support, and you spent countless hours with me talking in circles about the intrusive thoughts I was experiencing. I believe in my heart that had you not been there and showered your love on me early on, I might not be here today. I am eternally grateful for you. To my father, thank you for being the man you are, rooted in your beliefs, but also kind and not quick to judge. You proactively reaching out to me to see how I was doing when you found out I was too scared to tell you what was going on meant more to me than you'll ever know. The way you and Mom have supported me has given me the strength to help others. To my sister, you seemed to effortlessly understand what I was experiencing the moment I told you. There was never an ounce of judgment, just pure encouragement and support. To this day, you are one of the first people to remind me that seeking help is the best thing I can do. I hope to always support you the way you've been there for me.

To Dr. Aureen Wagner and Dr. Jonathan Abramowitz, when I showed up at your doorsteps, I was defeated. I was lost, scared, depressed, suicidal, and anxious. You both got me on the right path by utilizing Exposure and Response Prevention. Through your clinical support, I was able to reclaim my life and in turn help others. You both truly changed my life.

To Christian Williams, besides my family and Kate, you were the first person I told. Something inside of me told me you'd understand, and you did. You never judged, but always listened intently. You sought to understand and never blew me off. At that time in my life, you filled my life with laughter and purpose. Between talking "cash" to each other and attempting to build our dream business, that time period is forever embedded in my heart.

To David Hurst and the Lawrence Township crew, thank you for listening, caring, and supporting me. We have a unique friend group. Although we rip on each other constantly, when it's time to rally, we show up full force. That love I will never take for granted.

To the rest of the Raleigh family, you know who you are. You are the ones I sat down at coffee shops with, in the oasis at the Cisco office and at each other's places, dreaming up how our lives would unfold. Those conversations gave me the courage to pursue my passions even when it felt terrifying.

To Michael Ayalon, 2018 was a pivotal year. You gave me the opportunity and the platform to share my story with college students and impact lives. You taught me the dos and the don'ts of the collegiate speaking market. You put your faith in me and gave me the confidence to believe that my story mattered and needed to be shared. I'm lucky to know you and grateful for your mentorship.

To Lindsey Alexander, you took a rough manuscript and guided me down the path this book needed to go. Your ability to kindly but confidently provide feedback and guidance is a blessing. Thank you for all of your help on this body of work. Without you, this book wouldn't be where it is today.

ABOUT THE AUTHOR

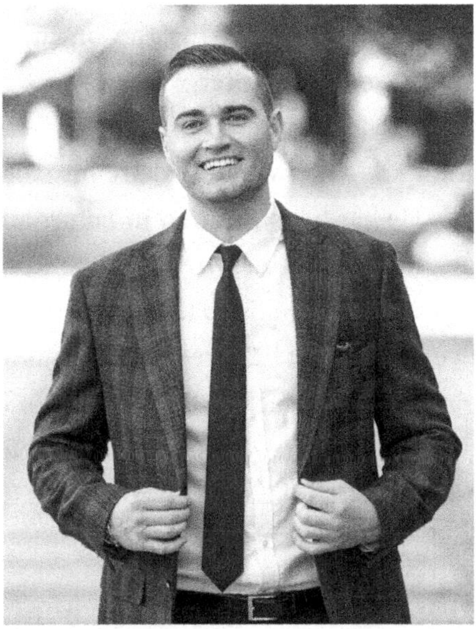

Zach Westerbeck is an engaging mental health public speaker, college success coach, and a certified Mental Health First Aid professional with a passion for helping college students and organizations understand the complexities of depression and anxiety in the modern world.

In 2016, he experienced crippling depression and anxiety for the first time in his life. During this period, he had thoughts of suicide and felt alone, scared, and unsure about his future. He suffered in silence for over a year before finally seeking help. This is why it is his mission to erase the stigma and normalize mental health issues by sharing his story with as many students and corporations as possible. His goal is to make the uncomfortable conversation around mental health comfortable in the hopes that it will save someone's life. Through his personal experiences, certifications, and extensive research, he is able to relate and clearly articulate why now more than ever it is critical to understand how to manage your mental health.

Zach graduated from Purdue University and is a brother of Sigma Chi fraternity. After graduation, he went on to work for Fortune 500 technology company Cisco Systems. He is the proud founder of Westerbeck Speaking and Coaching Inc., an organization focused on providing hope and resources for recovery for those struggling with their brain health. Zach has partnered with organizations like the Peace of Mind Foundation and One Mind to share his story and free those suffering in silence. He has been featured in *Forbes* and *Thrive*, among others. In addition, he has done interviews and podcast interviews with One Mind, the Peace of Mind Foundation, and the Freddie & Alyssa Show. He has spoken in front of hundreds of students at higher learning institutions and organizations such as Penn State, Chico State, Gamma Alpha Omega, UC San Diego, New York Institute of Technology, Georgia Tech, and University of La Verne, to name a few.

Web: zachwesterbeck.com
Instagram: @zach_westerbeck
Twitter: @Zachwesterbeck
LinkedIn: Zach Westerbeck

SPEAKING AND COACHING

Zach is available for speaking engagements as well as individualized one-on-one coaching for college students. His engaging, dynamic, and fun workshops are best suited for university students, college Greek communities, corporate wellness events and initiatives, keynotes, and nonprofit events pertaining to mental wellness.

To inquire, please visit zachwesterbeck.com/speaking or zachwesterbeck.com/coaching.

Made in United States
North Haven, CT
02 December 2021

11868821R00104